HOPES&
fears
DREAMS&
tears

HOPES& *fears* DREAMS& *tears*

a county memoir
NIRAJ MEHTA MD

PUBLISHED BY

MD2B
HOUSTON, TEXAS
www.MD2B.net

Hopes and Fears, Dreams and Tears: A County Memoir
is published by:

MD2B
P.O. Box 300988
Houston, TX 77230-0988

www.MD2B.net

ISBN # 978-1-937978-03-7

Library of Congress Control Number: 2014959443

Printed in the United States of America

For my indigent patients whose eyes fill me with Hope

For my teachers who helped me overcome my Fears

For the students and doctors who dare to have a different Dream

For Sheila, Natasha, Poonum, and Nikhilesh who wiped away my Tears

CONTENTS

ACT I: Medical School Years

ACT II: Residency Years

Intern Year

ACT III: The Attending Years

INTRODUCTION

Every fourth day, I have the same routine. I pull up to LBJ Hospital, aka "The County," to round with my post-call team at 5:45 a.m. Because the hospital will later become organized chaos, I bask in the peace and serenity surrounding me in the early morning dawn. Parking in the faculty lot, I chuckle knowing that the reserved spots will be mostly occupied by non-faculty members in the next three hours, and the rest of the parking lot will be a gridlock of illegally double-parked cars.

As I enter the side door, eyes of uncertainty meet me as a motley crew of patients waits for the business office to open at 6:00 a.m. for day surgery check-in. Given the large Hispanic patient population at LBJ, I used to start with my best Taco Bell Spanish greeting of "buenos dias." I abandoned that idea when my sincere but obviously ineffective effort led to more questions annunciated at one hundred miles an hour, no match for my mind which was translating at thirty miles an hour. Even when the breakfast of all doctors, coffee, kicked in, I could barely reach the speed limit when I translated Spanish in my head.

My eyes already had the deer-in-the-headlights look as I politely smiled back at the rapid-fire questions. I suddenly realized why Hispanic patients always seemed to stop me to ask for directions. Although my double-gelled Andy Garcia hairstyle and skin color seemed to offer an instant connection, they failed to realize that my outward appearance did not match my extremely limited Spanish vocabulary. Now, a simple "good morning" seems to do the trick of "beginning the day with a friendly voice, a companion non-obtrusive." (From my favorite band, Rush, and their song "Spirit of the Radio") Or does it? My mind begins to wander for a bit as transient idealism sets in as I approach the elevator doors. Another one of The County ironies: all three elevators work only when there is hardly anyone there.

As the elevator doors slide open on the fourth floor, I take a right turn to my office, looking forward to gently inserting the key into the door that leads to my heart and my soul. The walk to my office is my daily Prozac. As Lao Tzu noted, "the journey of a thousand miles begins with a single step." So it seems as I reflect on my last twenty years at LBJ, slowly taking baby steps towards my office each day.

As I walk, I see a nervous medical student. He is so focused on acquiring knowledge that he fails to realize he has the most precious of gifts—the ability to heal with his heart. I see a resident with a forlorn look. In his desperation to find light at the end of the tunnel, he has somehow lost himself. I wonder why doctors see The County as a stepping stone to greener pastures, thus choosing to leave, and why patients who end up at The County really had no choice.

Having almost come full circle and the time quickly approaching 6:00 a.m., I see the reflection of an attending physician who has not only survived in this environment, but finally appreciates The County for all its hopes and fears, all its dreams and tears. What an interesting idea for a …

ACT I

Medical School Years

The Age of Information

"I'm not dumb. I just have a command of thoroughly useless information."

Bill Watterson

1

Internal Medicine

We're so smart, we speak in riddles.

July 1, 1991. The day every medical student yearns for was finally here. We were starting our clinical years, the rotations that would ultimately help us choose a career pathway. This was true of most medical students, anyway—except that lame student who knew in kindergarten that he or she would grow up to be a left maxillary sinus specialist of thirty-two-year old Caucasian women whose last name began with the letter *B* (and perhaps ended with a *t*). Now there would be no more Krebs Cycle to memorize! No more looking for *ora serrata* on your cadaver! Yes, the best years of our medical school were about to begin.

I was nervous and excited to begin at the local county hospital, Lyndon B. Johnson (LBJ) in Houston, Texas. Unlike the third-year students starting similar rotations in today's medical schools, I had no orientation. I was told to report to 3C where the "team will explain the rest." So I jumped into my blue Nissan 200SX convertible, an upgrade from the scooter I'd had during the first two years of medical school, and took US-59 North to The County.

I'd lived in Houston since 1979, but had never been to this part of the city for reasons that would soon become obvious to me. As I approached LBJ, I realized that I was no longer in middle-class Houston, such as Alief on the southwest side, where I was raised. Instead, I was in the middle of mom and pop shops, small grocery stores, and what appeared to be fast food heaven. Only years later would I realize that the so-called McDonald's heaven was leading my patients at LBJ to a faster hell.

I saw more motorized scooters and wheelchairs than I could count and wondered if I was at Wal-Mart. Although every gate leading to the hospital parking lot was open, it seemed that every space was full. I would learn later that unless you arrived by 8:00 a.m. (something I would do consistently for the next seven years, even if I was running two hours late), there would be no parking spaces—you would be left to do laps in your own Indy 500, competing for the space that would hopefully vacate at the exact right time. After doing my own AJ Foyt routine for thirty minutes, I hopped out of the car and approached the seemingly harmless building with my short white coat—long coats were worn by doctors, and I wasn't one quite yet—and an overnight bag.

I was assigned to Team B, who happened to be on call that day. What luck! On the first day of my third year of medical school, I'm on an internal medicine service team that was on call! I didn't know anything yet, though. What would I do?!

I asked directions for 3C, and was told to take the elevators up and ask again. "Oh, by the way, only one of the elevators is working, so you might want to take the stairs, but I'm not sure which doors are open on which floors."

Where was I? Afraid that I might get lost if I used the stairs, I waited impatiently for the elevators, which patiently arrived fifteen minutes later. When I finally reached the third floor, I fumbled my way to 3C, wondering why Team B rounded on C. As if to feed my dry sense of humor, I almost collapsed—internally, of course, since I didn't want to be admitted to a county hospital after fainting—from laughter as the resident stated that B would usually meet on A, but not to confuse 3A with 4A because post-call we would start on 3C. Was he making this up just to mess with my mind?

We received our so-called formal introductions at this time. I quickly assigned a nickname to each member of the group, a skill that has served me well even to this day. The lead resident was from India and had a mustache that matched the one made famous by my favorite Indian movie actor. *Did I really say that? After all the years of torturing my parents by criticizing Indian movies, had I entered a parallel universe? Should I have taken the parallel hallway to the left instead of the right?* I naturally named him "Stache." One intern had a nose bigger than mine, which was no small feat, so I named him "Senior" since I was now officially "Junior" (thank God). This would create confusion because I would at times spit out "Senior," and Stache would turn around instead.

I wasn't sure what to do with the other intern until he began to speak. He had a very thick accent and was from Vietnam. I decided to call him "Morning" after *Good Morning Vietnam*. This moniker led to even more confusion because, at times, I would say "Morning," not always under my breath, at 11:00 p.m.

Finally, we were introduced to our attending physician, often called just "attending." The first thing I noticed was his age. I called him "Harvard," having been told that he graduated from "the med school beast in the east" in 1938. Now that I was standing in front of Harvard, I wondered if my friend meant 1838. This is when Harvard spoke to us for the first time. *Are you kidding? Was this guy a plantation owner? Was Lincoln still the President when he graduated?* I later learned that Harvard was from Charleston, South Carolina and had been a big shot at a medical school in "Carolinaahh" before coming to Houston. I would realize only much later the importance of what I learned during the introductions that day; there is no substitute in medicine for the power of humor and observations.

My first month at The County on an internal medicine service would be my first step on a journey I didn't know I was embarking on at the time. Since this was July, I learned later that the interns only one day earlier had been students, and that by extension (no pun intended in spite of the length of the worm under his nose) that Stache had been an intern. At least two things were working in my favor. Harvard had clearly been an attending for a long time, and more importantly, I wasn't the patient. I was told to leave my things in the call room and report to the EC. This was my first introduction to initials and abbreviations that I would continue to learn on the fly. The only things that weren't abbreviated in the chart, and especially during senior/junior conversations, were curse words. Or did "SOB" in the chart mean something else?

I came to the emergency room (ER=Emergency Room, EC=Emergency Center, both being one and the same) where I was assigned my first patient who—surprise, surprise—didn't speak a word of English. Morning told me that before things became even busier, I needed to see this patient with melena.

"What?" I asked.

"He has a GI bleed," responded Morning.

"Huh?" I continued with a look of confusion.

"He has a goddamned ulcer!"

Oh, sort of like the one I'll probably have by the end of this rotation! I said to myself.

"What do you want me to do?" I continued out loud.

"Well, he's Vietnamese, and I'm too busy to translate for you, so just go and tilt him."

I was too proud—or perhaps too terrified—to ask for help. I had no idea what "tilt" meant, at least not in the context that Morning meant. So, I approached the patient, who had a tube in his nose draining material that looked like ground coffee, and shook his hand. This was when the comedy of errors began. I started to shift the patient on his bed from side to side, in essence tilting him like I had been asked. I immediately felt as if a laugh track had been turned on for a live taping of *Happy Days*. The entire ER staff, which had been tense only two minutes earlier from what appeared to be a *M.A.S.H.* unit of endless patients, was on the floor, laughing uncontrollably after witnessing my ridiculous act.

Thirty days and counting, I said to myself as Morning, between bouts of humorous tears, showed me how "tilt" meant orthostatic hypotension, and how to correctly assess the patient for this important sign. I was crushed, but I'd made my first therapeutic intervention without realizing it.

When Morning translated what had just transpired to the patient, the seventy-plus-year-old-man with one tube, two IVs, and three concerned family members at his bedside, burst into laughter. It was my first honors grade as an MD-to-be, and like most other such rewards on this journey, it was only with time that I was able to appreciate its true meaning.

After a sleepless night of continued mishaps, I saw my first patient (Mr. Tilt) at 7:00 a.m. two hours before rounds with Harvard. The patient was now on 3C, but something was clearly wrong. He tried to communicate with me, but I couldn't make out what he was trying to say. Alarm bells in my mind were starting to match the butterflies in my stomach. I asked Senior for help. He was frantically preparing for rounds and in no uncertain terms told me, "Go away—it couldn't be that important." I ran to Morning for assistance and was told, "He can't speak English, nothing is wrong." I tried to tell him that the patient doesn't speak English, but now I wasn't sure if he couldn't speak at all because he was gesturing. There were no family members present, and I didn't know what else to do. Stache was nowhere to be found because, as the interns told me, "He's getting his ass kicked in morning report and whatever you do, don't page him."

Frustrated, I gave up until rounds. I presented the story to Harvard, leaving out, of course, the details of the tilt episode, and noticed that Harvard was smiling. I told him that something had changed that morning but I didn't know what it was. Harvard kept smiling. I told him that the patient had been talking yesterday and now I wasn't sure if he couldn't talk or didn't want to talk.

Harvard kept smiling and asked, "What else?"

Without trying to be funny, I stated, "The end."

At this point, Harvard turned crimson red and lifted the patient's right arm. To my surprise, the arm fell back onto the bed.

"My God, Niraj, this man has had a goddamn stroke involving his speech-dominant left hemisphere, and all you can say is 'THE END!'"

Since crap rolls downhill and I was at the bottom, I chose not to tell Harvard that I had run this by Senior and Morning, both of whom had dismissed my concerns and told me not to disturb Stache. I thought I would be perceived as a team player for falling on the proverbial sword, but I was wrong. I received the blame for not presenting information to the team in a manner that would have alerted them to the disaster. I learned another lesson that day. No matter what, the lowest rank receives the blame and the higher-ups are not held accountable. I would hope to change that someday.

You would think that the story of Mr. Tilt would end there, but it didn't. Usually when the proverbial you-know-what hits the fan as it did that morning, it's only the beginning. Why? We live in a society where someone must pay for the bad things that happen, and anger from family members can lead to litigation. As it turned out, one of the family members was a doctor who lived in another city. *What was the father of an MD doing at a county hospital?* I still haven't found a clear answer to that, even today, because I haven't seen another family member of an MD since that day at The County.

So what came next? Yes, you guessed it: a lawsuit. And yes, the family sued everyone who remotely had contact with the patient, including the medical student—me—who had nothing to do with the outcome. Once the lawyers found out who did and didn't have money, I was dropped from the lawsuit. I still remember the sick feeling I experienced when I was handed the subpoena, and I'm sure that my heart was probably visible in my mouth. I wrote to the best of my ability about my role—or lack thereof—in the care of the patient. I haven't been sued since that day, but as Tears for Fears suggested "Memories fade, but the scar still lingers." The litigation process is fraught with emotions for both physicians and patients. In the end, there are no winners, just losers with lost or broken lives that will never be the same.

I continued to excel at my deficiencies throughout the month, but at least I was consistent, for I knew nothing. I missed a Grade V tricuspid regurgitation murmur that Harvard claimed he could hear while driving home from work. Morning told me to read about the antibiotic vancomycin "pig and trough" and was upset the next day when I told him I could find nothing on the topic. I'd forgotten about his accent—I was supposed to look up "peak and trough" as it applied to the dosing of vancomycin. Senior continued to scold me about my lack of knowledge in neurology—the field he'd chosen, of course. I was called a "smart ass" (*but you just said I know nothing!*) when I reminded him that my knowledge was lacking in all fields of medicine equally, not just neurology.

With all my shortcomings, what was I good at? I didn't know then how important it was, but I spent as much time as I could with my patients. I would watch TV with them. I would follow stroke patients, including Mr. Tilt, with the therapist and even take them outside the hospital for a walk and a conversation, if they spoke English. I didn't understand why an eighty-four-year-old guy with lung cancer and end-stage emphysema couldn't smoke, so I would take him outside to smoke a cigarette. I would drive the team crazy by reminding them that another family member wanted to talk about their loved one. These requests inevitably came at the end of a long day because most family members worked and could only visit at night.

I would feed patients breakfast if they needed help. And most importantly, I couldn't understand death, and the twin lakes on my face would routinely flood over when a patient would die. Without realizing it, I was learning how to take care of people, not just their diseases. *Hopes, fears, dreams, and tears...*

I never received a Harvard education, and maybe that's why I never understood Harvard, the attending. Was I alone? There was a generation gap—or in this case, maybe a century gap—but Harvard spoke in riddles and analogies that I just didn't understand. From the chuckles I heard from other team members, I knew I wasn't the only one. One day, Stache asked if 40 milliequivalents of potassium chloride infusion administered intravenously (IV) over four hours was reasonable to correct a potassium value of 2.5 in a patient admitted the night before. Harvard responded with, "Am I my mother's keeper?"

Harvard's notes were just as ambiguous. An eighty-two-year-old patient was admitted with a heart attack and Harvard's note stated, "This man's children don't love him. Life is just not fair!" We were going over Killip classification (a system used to risk stratify heart attack patients) with Senior, and meanwhile Harvard was worried about love! Years later, I realized that Harvard's language had meaning, but back then, we were only hearing, not listening. Harvard wasn't his mother's keeper because part of residency was a learning curve of making mistakes—hopefully not catastrophic ones. What else could be more important at age eighty-two, after having lived a full life, than the love of your dear ones, especially after a heart attack? I chuckle now thinking of how history repeats itself, because my students now wonder why I speak in riddles. In time, they'll understand.

Finally, the last day of the rotation arrived, and it was time for me to receive my grade for the month. I had been dreading this day for some time. I was great at getting "informal honors" from patients, but the actual grade was a different story. Harvard sat me down in his office and started with yet another analogy. "Niraj, a few of you medical students need to be taken out to the parking lot and shot!"

I'm so tired of having a heart in my mouth, and it's only the first month of my third year! I thought.

"What do you mean?" I said sheepishly.

"Nothing personal, Niraj. Some of you are bright, but you're just not cut out to be doctors. You shouldn't waste time and we shouldn't waste time. You should just be shot and if you survive, go onto other things."

At this point in the conversation, I think my heart was trying to exit my mouth at the same time that something else was getting ready to exit the other orifice.

"Don't worry—you don't need to be shot!" Harvard went on.

How kind of you, I thought.

He continued, "There is a smaller portion of medical students that don't need me because you guys are too damn smart!"

Me, really? You're too kind.

He must have been a mind reader like Diego in *Ice Age* and immediately retorted, "No, you're not one of them."

I wondered what would happen if Harvard had a heart attack at that moment. I just wondered. Is that wrong? After all, I thought I was having one! Karma, right? C'mon, I'm Indian. These thoughts are natural.

"Then there are the rest of you, and that includes you, Niraj. You just started and you don't know shit, but you will get better with time. So you get a PASS."

By this time, I was a babbling lunatic. I shook his hand and said something to the effect of, "Stache, Senior, and Morning are at fault!"

To my amazement, he was about to start another analogy but the sound of his pager saved me. I left the fourth-floor office and ran to the nearest bathroom, which was being cleaned. Doing my best Ben Johnson—ok, let's make it Usain Bolt—I headed for another restroom on the third floor, but the elevator was delayed. Pissed off, almost literally, and having no other choice, I took the stairs. Thank God the door was unlocked.

The third floor bathroom was out of order, too. So I went straight to the patient's bathroom, and while contemplating on my PASS grade, realized that more than one Niagara Falls existed. Harvard was right—grade inflation in medical school is rampant, and attendings who give passes face a backlash, unless they went to school in 1938. How do I know? Today I mostly give passes and stick out like a sore thumb every month. Honors must be earned, not given, or else they have no meaning. I also discovered that the closest bathroom is always the one in the patient's room, and Murphy's Law exists everywhere. Perhaps Murphy worked at LBJ, and his ghost still roams the bathrooms.

2

Obstetrics & Gynecology

Catchers, beware of your balls!

Since I wasn't one of the chosen few who entered medical school with a preordained career choice (remember the maxillary sinus specialist?), I kept an open mind as I moved from one rotation to another. If I had time to think, perhaps I would have realized that internal medicine was The One for me. But there was never time to think in medical school, especially during the third year. So onward I went to the next rotation: OB/GYN, once again at LBJ. By now, I was Mario Andretti (who needs AJ?) and knew all about bathrooms, stairwells with unlocked doors, and working elevators. What could go wrong? Having no Stache, Senior, or Morning was icing on the cake. Well, be careful what you wish for, as they say, because…

At LBJ, OB/GYN, short for Obstetrics and Gynecology, was located on the second floor. *Why do people take elevators for one floor, anyway? Take the stairs! Assuming the door isn't locked.* Unlike internal medicine, OB/GYN was a hands-on rotation from day one. OB/GYN doesn't like to be known as this, but I quickly decided that they were simply surgeon wannabes.

On day one, I met the usual suspects and continued to assign nicknames to my superiors. That part was easy; it was obvious who gave and who took orders. The senior residents were gods and the interns were peons. It made me wonder what they thought of me. Oh, yes, the attending. Almost forgot. Let's just call him the Guitar Man because he actually brought a guitar to rounds on call days.

After brief introductions, I was told to follow a Peon. Within an hour, I knew that OB/GYN was not for me. There I was in the Operating Room (OR) with Peon catching "a gift" from God—the real God, not the senior resident. Or so they say. Maybe "a gift" is in the eyes of the beholder. It felt as if I was reliving my Little League years, once again playing the role of catcher. Didn't they always put the crappiest player as catcher? I had my booties (was I on the moon?) and my hat (actually a hairnet that made me look like the cafeteria worker). And of course I had the gloves (I thought it was a catcher's mitt). What was I supposed to do now, standing in the room with a pregnant woman? Peon told me to catch the baby. "No matter what you do, don't drop it" he said.

This triggered memories of the 1978 Little League Championship Game in Indiana. I remember a passed ball on a called third strike. I was the guilty catcher. As Yogi Berra had suggested decades earlier, this was going to be déjà vu, all over again. *Wait, wasn't Yogi a catcher too?*

"What will we be doing?" I asked Peon.

"Don't ask questions—just do as I say!" he retorted.

"Yes, sir, drill sergeant," I spoke under my breath.

Peon told the mother to push, or as I learned at LBJ, "*empuje.*"

That day, I caught my first slime-covered gift at 10:11 a.m. Why do I remember the time? Boy Genius here forgot to remove his watch. As luck would have it, some of the baby goo leaked past the glove onto the watch. While my classmates were excited and tallied the number of babies they delivered, I kept count of the number of days remaining in my OB/GYN rotation, keeping "hope alive" for the rotation to end long before it would become a catch phrase.

As was the case on Internal Medicine, trouble continued to follow me on OB/GYN. On the second day of the rotation, I was told to examine a pregnant patient. During pregnancy, the cervix generally remains firmly closed until labor, when it then begins to dilate. I was given instructions to examine the cervix for dilation, and report the findings to Peon. Next to each patient's bed was this ridiculous board which we could use to determine the degree of cervical dilation. By placing our fingers apart on the board, we could estimate how dilated the cervix was; we were taught to spread our fingers until we were touching the lateral walls of a patient's vagina.

What was this? Show and tell? I examined the patient and told Peon the os (opening of the cervix) was closed. He shifted his attention to other patients, since a closed os meant that, although the baby was on his or her way, labor was still in its early stages.

Thirty minutes later, however, god was screaming at me. That would be the wanna-be-god, the senior resident on the service, not the real God. Well, actually he was screaming at Peon. "How could this woman be completely dilated and we let her sit around to dilate?"

As it turned out, I couldn't feel the walls because the patient was completely dilated! Since I couldn't feel anything, I thought the cervix was closed. I thought I'd felt the cervix, but maybe I couldn't reach it because my fingers were too short. When you assume the cervix is closed wrongly, Peon's mouth is open widely. *An inverse relationship! There really is math in medical school.* He gave me a tongue lashing, the likes of which I'll never forget. The uvula in his mouth looked like a cervix winking back and forth in a vertical plane, and I couldn't tell if it was open or not.

I guess crap rolls downhill no matter which rotation you're on. I quickly learned that there are no stupid questions, and to always ask if you're not sure—even though you'll likely be admonished or ridiculed, especially on the surgeon wannabe rotations like OB/GYN. I also realized that people like to pass the buck, and no one likes to take the blame. More importantly, it was rare to find someone who loved to be with medical students and actually teach them. Someday, when I became an attending, I hoped to do better.

OB/GYN and I were like oil and vinegar, not mixing very well at all. A considerable portion of our time was spent in surgery but it was painfully obvious that I didn't belong in the operating room. In fact, I stuck out like a Yankee fan at Boston's Fenway Park.

By the time I usually reached the OR, the scheduled patient was heavily sedated under general anesthesia. Most of us had never talked to the patient. And yet, we would all perform pelvic exams to palpate the "abnormality," starting with the senior resident and working our way down the pecking order until everyone had taken a turn. I did this for two months, and my level of uneasiness grew every time. Did the patient consent to multiple exams, especially under general anesthesia? Was this OK because the consent form stated, "Dr. Guitar et al.?" Did the patient have any idea what "et al." meant? I hadn't done enough exams to understand what abnormality I was supposed to be feeling anyway.

Sadly, I never spoke up in these situations. Although there is no "I" in "team," all members of the team must feel free to voice their opinions. Was there such a thing as informed consent? How informed were our patients? Idealism ran through my bloodstream, and I even shed tears in the call room. Dreams and tears are sometimes lonely partners in life.

I also discovered the "six-inch rule" on the OB/GYN rotation. Having been raised in what is arguably considered "the chest capital of the South," I thought I knew exactly what the six-inch rule meant. And like everything else I assumed during my third year of medical school, I was wrong.

That day, I was the catcher once again at the base of the bed of a patient about to deliver another slimy slider. The patient was in excruciating pain, even though she was receiving IV pain meds. Peon was at the head of the bed, and during this particular encounter, playing the part of the patient's coach. He kept screaming at the player—I mean at the patient—and thank God, for once, not at me, "Push harder! You're not even trying!"

I guess the patient had had enough. She grabbed Peon's family jewels and squeezed as hard as she could, screaming, "I need more goddamned pain medications now, you little shit!" (Maybe I should have nicknamed Peon that instead, come to think of it.) Suddenly Peon, who had always been proud of his best low-pitched Lou Rawls voice, turned into Michael Jackson. He literally "Beat It" out of the room, and the lesson of the six-inch rule was indelibly etched in my mind: Never get within six inches of a delivering patient's hands at any time. Personally, I would make it at least a foot, to be on the safe side. The fear of those six inches remains engrained in my head even today.

The best part about OB/GYN, other than that it would come to an end some sweet day, was the Guitar Man. Here he was in charge of controlling surgeon wannabees, constantly surrounded by chaos, and yet he never became angry. He would run back and forth between three cases, always remaining in control.

On one particular occasion, both God and Peon were busy with a routine delivery. There was no one else available to catch the baby. Guitar Man looked at me and calmly spoke:

"Are you ready to assist me with this routine delivery?" I don't think the Guitar Man realized that there was no such thing as routine when I was involved. After talking to the patient, the Guitar Man told me that he would be right back. Although I had never been in the delivery room alone, he told me to get started. After all, it was nearly the end of the month and I hadn't dropped a baby yet.

I had just done my best Thurman Munson when Guitar Man walked in.

"Where are your booties?"

I looked down and saw uncovered Nike shoes, Air Jordans, by the way—black with red stripes. *Oops!*

"Where is your hat?" he continued.

Double oops. I thought I would surely receive a spanking to rival the one I received from God and Peon. Instead, Guitar Man simply stated a fact: "You're not going into OB/GYN, are you?" And he walked out.

I guess he realized the only perfection in training is imperfection. He later told me during my evaluation that the most important gift I had was the willingness to learn, and more importantly, to truly care about my patients in other ways, even if I wasn't interested in OB/GYN as a career. I felt like a fraud for not telling him about my uneasiness with doing pelvic exams on patients under general anesthesia. I promised myself that I would always speak my mind from that point forward. This would prove to be both a gift and a curse for me, as you will learn later. The coup de grâce of this story? OB/GYN was my only honors rotation during the third year of medical school.

3

Surgery

My life sucks and so will yours.

Can you hear the theme music to *Jaws*? Close your eyes just for a second and start humming it. Yes, there was blood in the water, and I was the victim: up next was the surgery rotation. Within the very first hour, it was obvious that this was a round-hole rotation and I was a square peg. This was the military, and I felt like Forrest Gump simply responding internally to all questions, "Yes, sir, drill sergeant." There were lots of rules. I called these rules my Surgery Top 10 List (see next page).

In spite of the Forrest Gump analogy, I couldn't name our chief "Lieutenant Dan." I called him BG for "Beyond God." I named the intern GWB for "God Wanna Be." The attending was named Stealth, for he was visibly invisible, especially during rounds, where BG ran the show.

Funny, I never really liked Internal Medicine or OB/GYN until I started Surgery. No more coat and tie: this was scrubs country. The best thing about scrubs—pajamas for doctors that usually come in different shades of green and blue—is that you could easily put on twenty pounds and never realize it.

SURGERY TOP TEN LIST

1) Surgery residents will never call you by name. I was "shithead" and my buddy was "dumbass."

2) Surgeons are right and you're wrong.

3) Unless you curse or have a strange cynical sense of humor, you won't fit in.

4) Attendings don't know you exist and couldn't pick you out of a lineup (more on this later.)

5) If surgeons get an inkling you're even thinking about going into internal medicine, the number of pimp questions will quadruple, and you'll be called a flea for sitting around and thinking too much. I'll let you guess what the flea is sitting on.

6) Surgeons will ask you only what you don't know. If you know Ranson's criterion for pancreatitis, they'll ask you who Dr. Ranson was.

7) Surgeons consider rounding on patients or doing anything outside the OR a punishment.

8) Your daily notes don't make any difference, and the estimated blood loss during surgery is always "minimal."

9) If you look up the word "cynic" in a Thesaurus, the word "surgeon" will appear first.

10) It took me years to understand this and I can't believe I'm actually going to say this. *(Did I take my Prozac? Am I delirious?)* Surgeons care very deeply, but no one should be subjected to the work hours that they were forced to manage (twenty-four hours on and twenty-four hours off). I believe this workload led to the aforementioned numbers 1 through 9 on this list.

The learning started from day one of the rotation. Lesson # 1: crap rolls downhill, and I was at the bottom of the pile. Stealth yelled at BG who yelled at GWB who in turn yelled at SH (Shithead = me). No matter what happened, it was my fault. Why did the "appy" (appendicitis surgery) go wrong? SH's fault. Why did the "lap chole" (laparoscopic gallbladder surgery) turn into "open chole" (open gallbladder surgery)? SH's fault. Why was it raining? SH's fault. Why did the Astros lose? SH's fault. I dreamed that someday all my fellow SHs and heads of teams would be on the same level.

I will never forget that surgery rotation. For the entire month, I didn't see a sunrise or sunset because I came to work early and always left late. Sadly, as hard as I was working, BG and GWB were working beyond human capabilities. Call for them was every other night; BG was basically on call all the time. What could GWB do without BG if a case came in and GWB was in house? Exactly! BG had to come to the hospital. BG worked so hard that I once saw him have visual hallucinations during rounds.

Stealth was there, but the volume of patients was so high that he had to be in multiple operating rooms at the same time. This was why he never recognized us peons. Our role was to serve primarily as the human retractor by keeping the abdominal cavity open during operations. We never spoke in the OR and wore masks and scrubs which kept our identities a secret. Yes, to Stealth, we were ironically visibly invisible. Who the hell was going to give us our grade for the rotation at the end of the month if no one recognized that we existed?

Why "ironically," you ask? Well, the four medical students on the rotation had no interest in surgery as a career. It was obvious that we were a convenient outlet for BG and GWB, a means to unload their anger and frustration over the unreasonable work hours they couldn't control.

So, we decided—yes, all of us—to call in sick near the end of the month and play golf at the Hermann Park Golf Course. On arrival to the course, I once again felt that heart-in-my-mouth sensation I had experienced during my internal medicine rotation. Why? Because Stealth himself was about to tee off, too! No, he hadn't called in sick. Attendings worked in shifts, and I guess this was his shift off. All four of us were in a state of panic, and I think that half our cardiac output directly went to our kidneys.

Before we could move, Stealth turned around and asked us where we went to school.

"Rice," I said.

"We hope to go to medical school," Dumbass continued.

"Shut up!" I said under my breath.

We thought for sure that this chance encounter with Stealth would be the end of us, but then the irony set in. Stealth really had no idea who we were, because in the OR we all looked the same and kept our mouths shut!

In fact, he even offered us $20 each to caddy for his foursome group. We declined, found the bathroom, and once again let a collective Niagara Falls perform its gravitational deed. We couldn't stop laughing for hours. Yes, we did finish the round. I shot a 62 on the front nine. What can I say? I couldn't concentrate, and besides I was never much of a golfer.

The surgery rotation was full of positives and negatives, but no other rotation stood out more during my years as a medical student. I remember a time when GWB was scolded by BG for stopping to help nurses with a patient.

"He is not ours," BG said, "and we're not carrying the code beeper! Move on!"

I also remember BG walking into a patient's room at 5:30 a.m., bluntly disclosing the diagnosis of colon cancer, and hurriedly leaving the room. At such moments, I was appalled by the lack of bedside manners and callous disregard for patients. The surgery rotation was a roller coaster of human emotions, one that demanded a "put up and shut up" attitude. We tried using humor to break the ice. Once GWB screamed at me, saying, "This is unacceptable, Dumbass." My friend intervened and said, "Sir, I'm Dumbass. That is Shithead." Even GWB cracked a smile. I think.

BG once asked me if I wanted to save lives. I quickly replied yes. BG told me that today was my lucky day and I would get to do exactly that.

I was excited and asked, "How?"

BG dryly replied, "I'm going to send you home early today."

The surgeons desperately wanted to be human and humane, but were instead forced into a robotic survival mode. I dreamed someday that the working hours would improve. That day arrived on July 1, 2003, courtesy of the Accreditation Council for Graduate Medical Education (ACGME), which formally mandated a maximum 80-hour work week for all residency programs. Although I passed the rotation, I would like to suggest that I merely survived it. After all, that should be the goal of medical school.

In reality, medical school most closely resembles fraternity and sorority hazing. Don't fear—just survive. It's ok to let the tears flow while keeping your hopes and dreams alive. Square pegs don't need to fit into round holes. They just need to look harder to find other siblings, equally desperate to find a home.

4

Pediatrics/Psychiatry/Family Practice

The Little Three with a big meaning

I don't mean to shortchange the Little Three of Pediatrics, Psychiatry, or Family Practice (although at the time I did), but those rotations didn't leave me with lasting impressions during medical school. Having just finished Internal Medicine, OB/GYN, and Surgery (The Big Three), something was just off with the Little Three. Looking back, it's possible that the Little Three failed to resonate with me because of location. I was not assigned to LBJ for these rotations and thus felt out of place. I had become accustomed to the constant adrenalin kick provided by the highly stressful and fast-paced environment of the Big Three. In contrast, the pace of the Little Three was slower and everyone seemed too nice. I wasn't used to the touchy-feely approach. What I failed to realize was that healing begins with feeling. I should have seen the Little Three as the Important Three rotations during medical school. Instead, my preconceived notions and lack of experience led me to draw erroneous conclusions about the Little Three.

Psychiatry reinforced for me the mind-body connection, although I didn't appreciate it fully until I became an attending. You would think that this concept would be easy for me to embrace, given that I was born in India. Sometimes we fight what we already know for no good reason, I guess.

Pediatrics taught me the value of a Shakespearean quote I would learn much later: "Let every eye negotiate itself and trust no agent." I couldn't figure much out during the pediatrics rotation because I felt as if moms and (rarely) dads provided their own Oprah version of the history. By the time parents had brought their child to the hospital or clinic, they already knew what was wrong and we were just there to take orders from Dr. Mom or Dr. Dad. Sadly, sometimes they were right and we were wrong and vice versa. At times, it was difficult to tell if we were treating the child or the caregiver. Given the subjective nature of the history provided secondhand by the parents, our differential diagnosis (possible medical conditions that could account for the patient's symptoms) seemed endless.

This often led to random tests. By "random," I mean parents asked why and the attending responded, "Because I said so." The results of these tests were at times even more confusing. What did we do to alleviate the "WTF" moment? We ordered more tests, which, more often than not, didn't change the child's outcome. This, however, led to a more important learning point: Kids are resilient, and like all other patients, at times they survive in spite of us—not because of us. Sometimes less is more.

Family practice provides nothing to me as a medical student, at least that is what I thought back then. And how wrong I was. That department, especially in a tertiary care medical center in Houston, was Cinderella, the stepchild of the medical school. Everyone laughed at Family Practice (FP) and assumed that if you went into FP, you weren't good enough to do anything else. Perhaps I felt that way because our FP rotations were in the community, and we hadn't been exposed to private practice settings on any other rotation except FP to date. Maybe the patients weren't sick enough and I, like all other med students, wanted an adrenalin rush.

In retrospect, though, family practice was the most important rotation of medical school. The Little Three were trying to impart wisdom, but I was too naïve to appreciate it at the time. The energy of youth outweighed the wisdom of age back then, I guess. These rotations, particularly Family Practice, were urging me to listen to patients and by extension their caregivers. My goal was to relieve human suffering, not just change lab values or numbers via transient and artificial interventions. How could we as medical students embark on such a noble, lofty endeavor if we didn't know how to listen to the sufferer?

My third year had come to an end, and T.S. Eliot's quote was constantly in my head, like an auditory hallucination that would not go away: "Where is the wisdom we have lost in knowledge? Where is the knowledge we have lost in information?" I guess I had the information, but, only with time, would I appreciate that knowledge alone was insufficient. Looking back, I hope and dream that students will be wise enough to recognize their fears, and more importantly, never forget their tears in learning to take care of patients, not just diseases. We may aim for a cure, but we should aspire to heal.

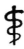

5

Fourth Year Medical School

What are you going to be now that you're grown up?

As every medical student knows, the most repeated question throughout medical school is "So, what are you going to go into?" The fourth year of medical school was decision time. The problem: I knew what I didn't like, but I wasn't sure what I liked. Surgery? No thanks—I liked sunrises and sunsets. OB/GYN? Yea, right. Might as well be a surgeon. Pediatrics? Seriously? I didn't care for the "Mommy knows best" baggage. Psychiatry? Are you crazy? I liked physical exams and at times wanted to tell patients to shut up. (Sorry, that's just me. Honesty is always the best policy.) Family Practice? I doubt it. I liked equal parts inpatient medicine and outpatient medicine. Besides, I'd always lived in the city and wouldn't consider moving to a rural community to practice FP the way I envisioned it.

Interestingly, the decision tree was sort of like a multiple choice exam question. I never memorized random facts, and thus never knew the correct answer. However, I could use my problem-solving skills to weed out incorrect answers and thus arrive at a reasonable conclusion as to the correct answer. Through a similar process of elimination, I chose Internal Medicine by default.

Now that I knew what I was going to do with my life—I guess that is the same as picking a residency—I had to separate the myths from the facts. Sadly, it was impossible to do so. Like all other Indian medical students—I'm willing to bet my life on the following statement—I was given unsolicited advice from my doctor "uncles and aunties" at Indian dinner parties. To those of you who are unfamiliar with the Indian culture, "uncle and aunty" simply means that my mom or dad somehow knows you! It didn't matter if the last time they talked to you was ten years or ten minutes ago. Either way, "uncle and aunty" didn't really know you from Manish or Himesh.

"Hi, Manish Beta, how are you? Uncle and I are so proud of you!"

"Uh, thank you, Aunty, but my name is Niraj," I replied politely, bringing out the bit of an Indian accent that was always necessary for this conversation. I had to humor myself since there was alcohol all around me, but unfortunately none to rescue me. All good Betas didn't drink in front of uncle and aunty.

"Oh, sorry, Beta, my fault. Uncle and I are doctors and we give so much advice because you know we've seen more Diwalis than you."

For those of you that are not Indian, "Beta" is the uncle and aunty version of "I think I'm supposed to know you from ten years ago—or is it ten minutes ago" and Diwali is the religious festival period just prior to the Indian New Year.

"Oh, man, not the Diwali line again. This isn't even an Indian movie," I said under my breath.

"Sorry, Niraj Beta. Speak up and don't be shy. Aunty couldn't hear you," said Uncle as he made his way to the bar for another Johnnie Walker Black Label.

"Sorry Uncle, my fault. I was just distracted. Please help me since you've obviously seen so many more Diwalis than me."

Where is my Phenergan for nausea when I need it? Shut up, voice, not now!

"Oh, Beta you're so kind. If Uncle and I had a daughter, you two would be perfect!"

Now I really thought I would throw up. I guess sometimes nausea does turn into intractable vomiting. I politely smiled and let her continue as another set of uncle and aunty approached us. *What is this?* I thought. *A competition?* I received all sorts of advice from the uncle and aunty conventions that I was a part of every other weekend during the fourth year of medical school. "Don't go into medicine, Beta, there's no money." *Really, then why do you have three Mercedes Benz, two kids in a private school, and an eight-thousand-square foot mansion with a pool?*

They never could understand why I so often chucked to myself during these conversations. "Make sure you specialize, Beta." *Why?* "Well, because you can't just practice general, and besides there's no money in general, Beta." *I thought you said there was no money, period. Now where is that bartender? Maybe I can sneak a couple of drinks and pretend it's Diet Coke. This Beta needs a drink.*

I was just glad that the topic of marriage wasn't broached by the second set of uncle and aunty (why didn't I invent Anti-Shaadi.Com! to somehow be a kryptonite force to repel all the constant pressures related to marriage, especially for aspiring Indian professionals). The most interesting part of our conversations: No one asked me what I'd like to do or my thoughts about becoming a doctor. I hoped that someday when asked for advice about career pathways, I would listen first and speak later.

Yes, the questionable factoids were rampant. Some of these even originated from your own medical school or current interns and residents who had attended other medical schools. "Make sure you only get letters from people with connections, because that's what matters." *I'm not opening a Patel Motel, for God sake.* "Interview at as many places as you can." *Will you pay for the travel?* "Don't go there—they said the program is unstable." *I'm still searching for the mysterious "they."* "Yes, but go where you'll have a better chance for a fellowship." *Did you consider I might stay in general medicine?* "They only take AOA (Alpha Omega Alpha, the national honor society for medical students) and they prefer MD-PhD." *Once again with the "they."* "The job market is not going to be there in the next few years." *I guess "they" said that too.* "It's cyclical, but you will be off cycle when you start out." *Stop smoking weed and take some English classes, for Pete's sake!*

Worse, it seemed like everyone, except for me, had a plan. Ironically, none of the plans were evidence-based. I dreamed that somehow I could eventually merge experience with evidence.

So what did I do? I went with my heart because my brain was short-circuited from too much information (a great song by The Police, by the way). Like the cable commercial says, I decided to "simplify." What did I value most? Location. Why? I had been in Houston since 1979 for one very important reason: I hated cold weather. Yes, I'm the guy who can't function below 60 degrees Fahrenheit. Just ask anyone who has ever known me. Unlike most people, I consider 90 degrees to be mild. In fact, I used to study under a tree in 95 degrees during college while the rest of my friends were in a library that, to me, felt like the frozen tundra.

Focusing on the weather was a good starting point because it eliminated many programs. I started by considering residency programs in the Southeast or the Southwest, including Houston. I liked the outdoors—biking and hiking—more than I enjoyed the water. Hum, sounded like the Southwest. If I decided to leave Houston for other programs in Texas, would I receive a better education? I believed and still do that the heart pumps blood the same way wherever you go, and it's what you do with the opportunities that matters. Besides, I was in the largest medical center in the world. If I was going to stay in Texas, Houston was the answer. Wow, that was easy.

I interviewed at my home base and added Phoenix, Los Angeles, and San Diego to the mix. Was this enough? I wondered. My friends were interviewing at no less than fifteen places. The only thing we have to fear is fear itself, right? (Say it with a British accent for effect.) Indeed.

6

The Interview Season

Extra scheduled days off

The interview season, was interesting, to say the least. I was required to obtain a letter of recommendation from the dean of the medial school as well as the Chairman of the Department of Internal Medicine. The dean clearly couldn't pick a particular student out of a lineup—unless of course that student had been in a *police* lineup during medical school. As to the chairman's letter? It was full of quotes and impressions from someone else's evaluations of me during the rotation. And how much time did these other people actually spend with me directly to form an opinion? I guess it was more time than the chairman had spent, but that wasn't saying much.

Of course, we were supposedly given a choice to waive our right to read the letter. I've never met a student that didn't waive that so-called right, but oh, how I wished I could've read those letters. During my interview circuit, I focused on my interviewers' facial expressions and other nonverbal clues (like a Bell's palsy smile or shifting in the chair as if suffering from an acute bout of tenesmus), hoping to discover some clue as to the contents of those letters. Did someone comment on my tilting skills? Or did someone find out about my Golf Tour de Hermann, which included the golf course but not the hospital?

Such was the dread of the interview season. Not knowing what they could've known was torture. Most of us weren't AOA (Alpha Omega Alpha, the honor society for "academically gifted" medical students) or future Nobel Prize winners. So how the hell would the interviewer separate me from the other Nirajs or Manish Betas of the world?

My ace in the hole would be the letters from the dean of the medical school and the chair of the department. On second thought, if I was relying on those letters, I might as well have put my head in a hole and waited for the sunlight to brighten my face. I think this is when my first understanding of water brash as a symptom of GERD (Gastroesophageal Reflux Disease, or heartburn) began, but twenty years later, for a variety of reasons is still going strong in my mouth.

So off to interviews I went. First stop: Good Samaritan Hospital in Phoenix, Arizona. Although I had no idea of anyone's qualifications, the candidates applying for residency looked great as a group. Everyone was in their dark suits or dresses, with not a hair out of place. Plastered on their faces were uneasy smiles. Was I at an Indian wedding or an interview? We came from the four corners of America with different backgrounds, all thinking the same things: *Isn't my interview sort of like a blind date? I've never met this person. What if I say the wrong thing? Am I supposed to say a lot or very little? Should I ask questions or will the intent be misinterpreted? Is the guy sitting next to me going to take the last spot at this program, MY SPOT, DAMN IT?*

My heart rate was all over the place, reflecting my level of anxiety. I would learn much later that this was a good thing. I walked into the office of the chairman (I'll call him Frank Reich, the former quarterback of the Buffalo Bills) and

I knew immediately that I had walked into a nightmare. I was surrounded by Buffalo Bills paraphernalia! Really? It was less than two weeks after the Houston Oilers (did I mention I'm from Houston?) had blown a 32-3 halftime lead against the Buffalo Bills in an NFL wildcard game. "Greatest comeback of all time" was one headline. "Choke City Houston" was another. I had seen the recap of the game on every local TV station, multiple national stations including the four-letter network, and heard enough venom from local fans on sports talk shows to make a cobra jealous. And here I was walking into the lion's den—or maybe the Buffalo's den.

The opening question from Frank was: "So, you're from Houston?"

Why don't you just inject the potassium chloride into my vein right now, for there is no call coming from the Governor, I was thinking. I politely replied, "Yes, sir."

"Do you like football?" he retorted.

Do you like buffalo wings? is what I wanted to say, but again I responded, "Yes, sir."

So, the slow kill went on for another thirty minutes as we—I use the term loosely—dissected the game. He seemed impressed and told me I would be a great fit for the program. *Really, so you could humor me to death every time you saw me?* I thought. *I am Hindu, maybe another life closer to returning as human? Mom claimed 84 million lives, allegedly. No thanks.*

I shook his hand, blitz-tackled him in my mind, and crossed out Good Samaritan Phoenix from my already narrow list of possibilities.

The rest of my interview circuit was not much better. The opening question at Scripps Mercy San Diego was about the Krebs Cycle! Are you serious? You might as well ask me about my plans to get pregnant. At least you would have gotten a smartass answer instead of what my mind was reciting at the time: *Frank Reich is not my hero. Frank Reich is not my hero.* I'm not sure what I mumbled, but I'm confident it wasn't impressive, for I saw Bell's palsy and acute tenesmus at the same time for the first time, but unfortunately not the last. *Was there an association,* I wondered? Same story, same ending, just a different day. Another handshake, another closing of the door.

Cedars-Sinai in Los Angeles was next, and it was just not for me. The tour of the program focused on the celebrities that were currently being treated there or had been treated at the so-called Hollywood Hospital in the past. All I could think of was Prince singing:

…So when you call up that shrink in Beverly Hills
You know the one, Dr. Everything'll Be Alright
Instead of asking him how much of your time is left?
Ask him how much of your mind, baby
'Cause in this life things are much harder than in the afterworld…

No, I couldn't see myself as Dr. Beverly Hills, so another polite handshake with a forced smile closed another door.

My final stop was Wadsworth VA Hospital in Los Angeles. It was like an old girlfriend. Or was I thinking of my current girlfriend back home, LBJ? Everything was familiar: the droves of patients, the overwhelmed system, and the inefficiencies that permeated every corridor. My senses were intoxicated with the aromas I was already familiar with. Chaos was everywhere. And yet, the hospital was full of life, full of people doing the best they could with the limited resources they had. Just like at LBJ, in all the words and all the actions, I sensed hopes, fears, dreams, and tears. Had I found a new home or was there only one true home for me?

I had saved my home base interview for last. LBJ was familiar to me, and after having been everywhere else, what could go wrong? For once, everything went fine. Murphy and his law must have been on vacation. Now that I interview candidates, I know that when your medical school grants you an interview, it's a simple gesture of politeness. Nothing more, nothing less. Yes, your medical school would like to hold on to you if you're outstanding, but doesn't want to make you feel inferior if you lack the qualifications. It's easier for the school to interview everyone and save the disappointment of rejection for a few months down the line. Sometimes I wish I didn't know now what I didn't know then. Either way, with the interview season now over, I was ready to submit the rank list.

7

Rank, Match, Graduate

Game, set, and match

Paranoia runs rampant in medical school, in no small part due to the presence of so many Type A (*I wonder if the A stands for not such a flattering word that reminds me of the Time Magazine headlines when Mount St. Helens erupted in 1980*) personalities. The paranoia was further heightened during the fourth year of medical school when students applied for positions in residency programs. The process culminated on Match Day, often in dramatic fashion, as medical students across the country learned of their fate at exactly 12:00p.m. Eastern Standard Time. To participate in the Match, students ranked their preferred residency programs in order of desirability. Programs were asked to do the same with their list of applicants. A computer would then match up the highest preference from each side and work its way down.

All kinds of questions, rumors, and speculations floated around the medical school. *How many programs are you going to rank? Did you know that John Hopkins didn't fill last year because they only ranked MD-PhDs? Should you go somewhere else or stay at your medical school? Did you send thank you notes to all of the interviewers or just the program?*

What if I have to scramble into a program (meaning nobody you ranked wanted you)? I wish there was a better term for the last question because my favorite dish is scrambled eggs.

Great, I said to myself as my mind started to wander once again, thinking about Yogi Berra's catch phrase. Memories of picking teams for street football during middle school resurfaced, a time when no one wanted the Indian kid. Would this turn out the same way? Wait, this would be worse. Now there were too many damn Indian kids that everyone wanted, and I was still "average," at least according to the dean of the medical school and the chairman of internal medicine. *Stay positive,* I told myself, as I tried to force my internal voice to shut the hell up and let me have a moment of hopes and dreams instead of irrational fears driving unnecessary tears.

In February, I ranked Houston first and Los Angeles VA Wadsworth second. The match results were announced in March, right around the Ides of March. *Great, that's just great. How many more people are going to mess with my mind, Brutus?*

"What, Niraj? Are you on drugs? You're only ranking two places? Are you out of your mind? What if you have to scramble?" said my friends. Please, not the eggs again. Even my friends seemed like my enemies. Or was I the one being illogical? Help me, Spock! Against conventional wisdom—or more correctly, any wisdom at all—I ranked only two programs and submitted my match list.

The day with the greatest heart rate variability in medical school is, in my opinion, not the day of the match. It's what may or may not happen several days before. This is the day when you went nervously to your school mailbox and hoped it was empty. If it had an official letter from the dean of your medical school, you died *(I'm one life closer to reincarnation again as human, Mom!).* The dean was always the first person to be notified if the medical student didn't match. The term "undesirables" comes to mind. *You were right, Dad: everything has to do with India.*

So, off to the mailboxes we went as a group. I couldn't believe my eyes, but there was a letter from the dean in my box! *WTF?* I rarely cursed, but there were moments when nothing else could capture the emotion like that one four-letter word. I had been rejected by my own school? And for internal medicine, which was not a competitive field, at least not at my medical school. Here arose the water brash again! Or was I having a heart attack? Could I have just ruptured my aorta? Or hell, I was probably dying from all of the above. Perhaps I was dreaming.

I looked at the letter again, and asked my friends to pinch me. They did, not so softly, and this was clearly no dream. I had to scramble *(again with the eggs)*, tell my Indian parents that their son was a failure *(I think I saw a Hindi movie with this plot, or was it a thousand Hindi movies with this plot)*, and would now forever be known as the untouchable from my class.

Laughter burst from my friends.

"You think this is funny? I thought you were my friend, Christian!" I said to my best friend in medical school, a devout Baptist girl.

"Well, you've been laughing at us for ranking too many places. And you've been bragging how you'll get in after ranking just two. So we decided to play a joke on you," she said.

I looked at the letter again and was still confused. "What the hell—oh sorry, I mean what the heck are you talking about?"

By now, others were laughing, and Christian explained. My friends had actually traced the dean's signature and used a variety of Photoshop techniques to create the fake "you suck" letter to dupe me into thinking that I didn't match. Although I went through multiple episodes of sudden cardiac death in my mind, during that fifteen-minute period, I was once again reminded of what is and isn't important. I was still alive, I still had friends, and if you laugh at yourself, others will join in. I began laughing, and my friends joined in once again until we all had tears. I guess some tears are sweet after all.

I graduated from medical school in 1993 without much fanfare, given my academic excellence—or lack thereof—in medical school. I had not made a *B* since my freshman year of high school. I thought I'd tell you that tidbit before you hear it from my parents and "uncle and aunty" who tell you about the smart Beta—or the smartass Beta. Once I reached medical school, however, I prayed early and often for *B's*. I wasn't junior AOA, senior AOA, or AOA waitlisted. Let's just say I wasn't AOA, the national honor society for gifted medical students. I finished in the middle of my class. I got an MD, which stood for Mostly Dangerous to your health, and my parents threw a big party. Yes, their son was a good Beta.

I had recurrent nightmares that my parents were getting ready to send me to India, and would thrust in my hands an additional one-way ticket for return to the United States (code words for "you're going to get married, Beta!") Little did I know then that my journey was just beginning and that LBJ was to become not only my journey, but also my lifelong destination. Why? I had matched at my home base program and would be staying in Houston for residency.

ACT II

Residency Years

Age of knowledge

"Real knowledge is to know the extent of one's ignorance."

Confucius

The first year of residency is known as the intern year, and nothing could have ever prepared me for this disaster—clearly not medical school, anyway. I had heard countless stories of physical and mental exhaustion, self-doubt and survival of the fittest, relationships falling apart, and even contemplation of suicide. I thought the days depicted in *House of God,* the 1970's cult novel describing life during residency, were long gone. As usual, I was wrong. How I wish the ACGME (Accreditation Council for Graduate Medical Education) would have enforced the eighty-hour work week starting June 24, 1993 rather than July 1, 2003.

8

Neurology

You're not smart enough to start on internal medicine.

In the summer of 1993, I started my internship on the Neurology service. As I would later learn, I wasn't "strong enough" to start on the Internal Medicine Ward Service and clearly not ready for the Emergency Room, Medicine Intensive Care Unit, or the Coronary Care Unit. This was code for "he might kill somebody."

Since I would spend the next three years in internal medicine, I didn't see the point of neurology, especially as my first rotation. I was able to simplify every rotation to its core value even during medical school, and neurology as an intern was no exception. Since I was on the inpatient neurology service, the bulk of my time was spent dealing with acute vascular disasters, including strokes. I distilled my neurology rotation in three days:

- If a patient came to the hospital with unilateral weakness that was presumed to be due to stroke, the Emergency Room doctor ordered a CT (Computed Tomography) scan of the brain.

- If an area was darker than usual on the CT scan, it represented a stroke, and Neurology would be called (me!).

- If the area was whiter than the rest of the surrounding area on the CT scan, which we deemed "hyperdense" to make us sound smarter than the rest of the world, it represented an intracranial bleed, and thus Neurosurgery would be asked to see the patient (yeah, not me!).

- If the patient's presentation or findings did not warrant a phone call to Neurology or Neurosurgery, call Physical Medicine & Rehab (PM&R, or as my neurology upper-level resident used to say, Plenty of Money & Rest).

Obviously, neurology is far more complex than my summary would suggest. After all, the 90s was the decade of the brain (further proof of my elephant memory). No matter what anyone tells you, I didn't sleep through all of my medical school lectures, just the majority. But for an intern, what I wrote above pretty much summarized it. I also learned that no one, with the exception of the neurologist, documented a good physical exam when it came to the neurology portion of the exam. Looking at the written physical exams on charts made no sense to me. It ranged from "technically difficult due to language barrier" *(why don't you call a translator?),* "mild weakness" *(I'm not sure if weakness is there or not),* "exam not consistent" *(because it is changing or because the examiner doesn't know what he's doing?),* and my favorite, "grossly non-focal" *(the exam wasn't really done or even attempted).*

It was disheartening to see how we relied so much on technology but spent very little time actually examining patients in detail. Sadly, we rarely tried to understand how someone who had been walking and talking forty-eight hours earlier now felt emotionally. Why did it seem as if I was the only one asking "how would you feel if suddenly you couldn't speak or move one side of your body?" There was no patient hand holding, and very little eye contact. Like robots, we identified the cause of the stroke, modified risk factors, and then moved on. If being human is to feel, then did being a doctor mean you have a Tin Man's heart? One day I hoped and dreamed that I would lead a teaching service that would emphasize healing with equal parts heart and mind.

$

9

Float Month

Pray for a visible upper-level resident

Neurology ended in a flash, and I was back at LBJ (the neurology rotation had been at another hospital) for the float month. There were four internal medicine admission teams at LBJ, and call was every fourth day from 7 a.m. to 7 a.m. the following day. This meant that the on-call team would admit new patients through the ER during that period. Since the other three teams were not on call during that twenty-four-hour period, they would check out their patients to me starting at 5:00 p.m. For the next fourteen hours until 7:00 a.m., I would be responsible on average for sixty patients. I would then go home to sleep and return at 5:00 p.m to do it all over again. What was my residency program thinking? I had just finished a neurology rotation and now this? I couldn't just order CT scans of the head on all my patients. We didn't even have a neurology service at LBJ. Neurosurgery? Are you kidding? That was available at the bigger brother of LBJ, a county hospital known as Ben Taub. If the availability of the first two services was a pipe dream, what do you think about the likelihood of a PM&R Service at LBJ? Forget about it.

The good news: at least in theory, I had an upper-level resident to help me. But that was the problem with residency: There was a lot of theory. In reality, there was one other float intern and two upper-level residents for the month. So, in theory, one intern and one upper-level resident would be in the hospital every night. After all, what would the intern do if help was needed? I was good for handling basic stuff like nausea or constipation, but not much else. I could also give people sleeping meds (so I could sleep), but I was suddenly scared that they might not wake up while I was fast asleep. The damn Gujarati guilt gene. I wish I could've spliced it out!

Unfortunately, as I would learn throughout residency and especially during the intern year, you don't get to choose whom you will work with. The program would pair strong/weak resident/intern combinations, but this method never took personalities or value systems into account, and as a result, disasters ensued.

One of my upper-level residents during the float month was moonlighting at the jail the entire time to supplement his meager salary. Every time I had a question, he would respond with theory-based answers, waxing on about preload/afterload or the Frank-Starling curve over the phone.

"But what the hell am I supposed to do?" I would bark. "Give him fluids, oxygen, diuretics, none of the above, all of the above, how much, how fast, how long?"

The louder and more desperate I sounded, the calmer he would get over the phone. I wished I could somehow have gotten my fist through the phone and given him my Rocky Balboa on the other end. I named my resident Stealth because he was visibly invisible the entire month. No, his dad wasn't an attending on my surgical rotation during medical school.

My other resident was more helpful, but he had a severe snoring problem. Let's just say the only way to wake him up was to repeatedly bang on the door to his call room.

He was immune to the sound of pagers, and I called him Narcosleepy for my own amusement. I remember a time when I was called by the nursing unit. A patient was turning blue. I ran over to the patient, who sure enough was looking more and more like the Indian god Krishna. I highstepped my way in record time to Narcosleepy's call room and pounded on his door. "You gotta help me. This guy is turning blue!"

I could never tell if Narcosleepy was being patient with me or if the CO2 retention from his sleep disorder caused him to be mellow. He rolled his eyes, and we hurried to the unit where the patient was located. Narcosleepy noticed a hissing sound. After having received a breathing treatment, for some reason, the patient's supplemental oxygen had come off and the mask was on the floor. Yes, the floor was receiving 50% oxygen rather than the patient. The hissing sound came from the flow of oxygen through the tube.

Narcosleepy rolled his eyes again, hooked up the oxygen, and the patient's color returned to normal. Lesson learned. Common sense is not so common, especially when you're an intern.

The month zipped by, and I don't think I killed anyone, but then again how could anyone be sure? I prayed and hoped that every patient that I had pronounced dead wouldn't suddenly wake up. *(No, Mom, he wasn't being reincarnated instantly from the good karma of a previous life)*.

On the last day of my rotation, as I was walking out of the hospital at 7:00 a.m., I ran into a guy I'd never seen before in the parking lot. "Thanks, man," he said to me.

I asked him if I knew him. He said I should have. I was talking to Stealth! I guess some things can't stay invisible forever, even at LBJ. My mind was dreaming of one day becoming Stealth. My heart was hoping that I wouldn't become the person I despised. I guess the heart and mind conflict lies within the struggles of doctors, too, just like in patients. In the end, would I want a bigger heart or a bigger mind? Time would tell.

10

CCU

Damn it, everyone has %$@##%* chest pain, including Momma.

Just survive, baby, just survive. That was my mantra going into the next rotation, the Coronary Care Unit (CCU). Prerounds with the cardiology fellow were at 4:15 a.m., which meant the interns came to the hospital at 2:30 a.m. to gather information on patients. Every story sounded the same: chest pain, shortness of breath, chest pain, shortness of breath. Our attending would meet with us at 6:30 a.m. for rounds and then disappear into the cardiac cath lab for the rest of the day. *How many Stealths were there in this program? Did his son just come off the float month at LBJ?*

This was also the first rotation where we took care of private patients—my first exposure to medicine as a big business. Private attendings rarely taught and just needed someone to babysit the patients during the day after a procedure. (Translation: "Intern, please admit and discharge this patient for me.") Yes, the system was already broken, even back in 1993.

The only saving grace for the month: the multiple bouts of humorous patient encounters. My first patient was an elderly woman from a nursing home. She looked like the lead character in the movie *Throw Momma from the Train,* and as such I labeled her Momma. It seemed Momma had a tremor that was somewhat exaggerated during sleep. The monitor alarms at the nursing home would erroneously register this tremor as a cardiac arrhythmia, specifically slow ventricular fibrillation. Since she was hard of hearing and slept peacefully, someone at the nursing home would call a code and shock her with an electrical current of 300 joules to try to get her slow ventricular fibrillation back to normal sinus rhythm. Interestingly, after you shock any patient, much less an elderly woman who is wondering what the hell is going on, the patient is prone to developing chest pain. As a result, Momma would come to the emergency room and be admitted to us for unstable angina, a term used by cardiology to suggest an impending heart attack.

Unbelievably, the emergency room admitted her to us twice in the same month! When we'd ask her why she was here, she would tell us, "Some idiot shocked me while I was sleeping." I didn't know whether to laugh or cry. I probably did both. Lesson learned: Never trust anything the emergency room tells you because taking a reliable history is not their strength. Lesson learned: Listen to your patients and they might tell you what's wrong with them. By the end of the month, I had learned that all doctors were capable of hearing, but few were actually listening. I hoped to change that someday.

11

Emergency Room

Welcome to hell.

I thought the cardiology rotation was bad, but a worse hell awaited me next. Now I knew why the ER never seemed to be able to take a good patient history. There was no time. Our ER shift at LBJ was twelve hours on and twelve hours off. It was like "déjà vu all over again" every day. *Damn it, Yogi, I'm a Yankees fan, but this is getting ridiculous.* I was starting to wonder if Bill Murray's *Groundhog Day* was meant to be about the ER.

Yes, I had returned to the infamous birthplace of the Tilt Incident during my medical student days. And yes, unfortunately the nurses remembered. You see, misery loves company, and the only way to survive was to make fun of something or somebody. In the ER, you saw everything and anything. Frankly, if you weren't there, it was hard to separate fact from fiction, and myth from reality. The ER is where I saw my first interesting clown tattoo. The two nipples were the nose of the two clowns.

The ER was where half the doctors dated all the nurses, or was it the other way around? Either way, it was easy to figure out because a nurse and a doctor missing at the same time stuck out like, well, like a clown tattoo with nipples for noses.

As a group of doctors in training, we saw so many laboratory abnormalities that we created the Lab Olympics. Our patients were the unknowing participants. In our lounge, we had a board where the gold, silver, and bronze winners for winning lab values were listed. The lowest and highest laboratory results that seemed incompatible with life were considered winners. I was sure none of the "winners" would survive. As usual, I was wrong. Remarkably, nearly all of our Olympic medalists survived.

I personally took care of the gold medalist for low blood glucose with a value of 1. I also admitted another gold medalist (what other color could he be?), a man with a bilirubin of 88. We bragged about our champion and expressed disappointment when our winner was bumped. "Did you see the new pH gold medalist? It's 6.74? What? Yeah, and he walked out of the MICU yesterday and is going home today." "Did you hear about the hemoglobin of 2 that walked in? Literally walked in! He said he was just feeling a bit tired."

I guess having a sense of humor that was clearly morbid at times was our subconscious means of survival. We also learned how to send patients home from the ER if we didn't think they needed to be admitted. For example, I was taught that all chest pain was reproducible if you pushed hard enough. Since reproducible chest pain did not suggest cardiac emergency, we would be able to send the patient home. I would learn much later that even reproducible chest pain could be a rare presentation of a heart attack.

We had the three strikes rule for the month. If I saw you three times in the emergency room the same month, you were a GOMER (Get Out of My Emergency Room, from the

House of Gods book). If you had more than one chart, you were also a GOMER. We even came up with the concept of frequent flyer mileage: once you reached a limit, congratulations! You won a free cab ride home again. We were so cynical that we didn't care that "home" sometimes was not accurate; some patients were homeless and lucky if they received a cab ride to a shelter.

We invented new terms like "patent pending." Many patients presented to the Emergency Room with extremely elevated blood pressure. It was not unusual to see values above 240 mm of mercury. Unfortunately, the manual blood pressure machine did not register values above 240. Above this value were the words "patent pending." So, if we couldn't manually compress the radial artery at the maximum level of cuff inflation to estimate the systolic blood pressure by palpation, we would call the Medical Intensive Care Unit (MICU) and tell them we had a "patent pending admission" (code word for hypertensive emergency).

We learned that a distended belly did not always suggest there was ascites (fluid in the abdominal cavity) that needed to be removed by inserting a needle, a procedure called paracentesis. I was relieved to not insert the needle on one particular instance. Why? Because lucky for the patient and I guess by extension me—I didn't want to see the subpoena papers from the lawyers again—the alleged ascites spontaneously resolved in the ER when the patient delivered a baby.

I saw Jesus for the first of many times that month in the ER. Actually it was a psych patient who never took his meds and always came to the emergency room claiming to be Jesus. I think my parents would have been happier if it was Ram, Krishna, Vishnu, or any of the other Indian gods I was supposed to remember from my time at Indian Sunday school. With so many patients in the ER claiming to be Jesus, I began to wonder if I was part of an Oliver Stone conspiracy theory movie. Was I being brainwashed in an attempt to convert me into Christianity? *(Stop worrying, Mom and Dad. I'm still Hindu.)*

I was exhausted by the end of the month, living on as many as ten Diet Cokes or cups of coffee per day, sometimes both, and eating unhealthy cafeteria food (nachos!) at 2:30 a.m. My colleagues and I learned by doing and felt as if Dante's circles were missing a layer called "LBJ Emergency Room." And yet somehow, for the first time, I felt as if I was actually saving a life. I guess BG from my surgery rotation as a medical student was wrong after all: I didn't have to go home early to save a patient's life, although I wished I could have gone home early just once during my ER rotation.

In the end, seeing the same patients and diseases again and again and making mistakes—learning was all quantitative with high volume and poor supervision—taught me that patients sometimes survive in spite of us, not because of us. Although the pearls of learning information varied by rotations and subspecialties, the principles of taking care of human beings were universal: Look at your patients first and the lab results second, for even dead patients may have lab results that can be transiently fixed. Sometimes the best medicine is watchful medicine. Ah, maybe being a flea wasn't so bad after all.

12

Days Off

Cynicism has come to stay.

By now, you might be asking, "What did we do with our time off?" A better question would be "Did we *get* time off?" The answer was yes and no. Yes, we had time off, but we were constantly pressured to take *less* time off. On average, the interns had two days off a month if they were lucky. This generally depended on whether or not you had a kind-hearted upper-level resident. Did I mention that a kind-hearted resident was an oxymoron?

Early in the intern year, we tried to complain about our concerns as a group. For example, we complained that prerounding with a cardiology fellow at 4:15 a.m. was unfair because it forced the interns to come to the hospital at 2:30 a.m. We also felt that space was lacking in the call room during our CCU rotation. Since we would complete our previous day's post call at 9:30 p.m., what was the point of going home for four measly hours? The team that was on call that particular day now used the call room. How could all of us get some shut-eye if there were more bodies than beds? Among our other concerns were lack of teaching from private attendings and spotty supervision on some rotations. The answer was always the same from the leadership hierarchy, regardless of rank or position: "I remember when I was a resident that things were much worse. You're very lucky."

"Really? So, you hated walking uphill through snow ten miles both ways so we should have to?" *Shut up, Niraj. Why do you always have to say what everyone else is thinking?*

"Yes. And what's your name, young man? You seem extremely passionate about this discussion." Translation: This conversation is over and you're now on our watch list.

Since venting led you to be blacklisted, after a while we learned to keep our mouths shut. What did we do on our day off now that we had extra time? Well, we thought about quitting, because no one cared. Somewhere along the way, my smile disappeared and tears frequently appeared for no reason—or too many reasons. The only constant is change, unless you were in residency in the early 90s. Then, the only change was the lack thereof.

Different people dealt with residency in different ways. Some quit, some drank, some used drugs, and some engaged in promiscuous sexual behavior. I became depressed and closed everyone off. Yes, the smile was indeed gone, replaced by the angry frown that not even the memory of clown nose nipples could take away. Medical school idealism was long gone and residency cynicism had set in. Lao Tzu may have been right in suggesting that the journey of a thousand miles begins with a single step, but I don't think he would have ever completed his journey if he was a resident at The County. Hope was gone. Dreams were replaced by nightmares. And in time, even the tears dried up. Fears? You must feel in order to have fears. I was becoming immune to any feelings and disgusted with what I had become.

13

Ward Rotation LBJ

Never Ass-U-Me!

I was back on the LBJ Inpatient Ward Service the following month, this time as an intern, and paired with a familiar attending. Yes, it was my old friend Harvard from Charleston. I asked him if he had shot any medical students this past year, but he just smiled. Was he deaf, did he have Alzheimer's, or was the shooting a secret I was supposed to keep?

My steep learning curve continued with humorous interludes. It was difficult to find a translator at LBJ, especially at night. Having taken three years of Spanish in high school and college, I thought I could make do with my limited Taco Bell Spanish. Who needed a translator? *"Yo quiero Taco Bell,"* my internal voice would say as I approached a Hispanic patient, assuming that the patient didn't speak English.

On a particularly busy call day, I started and completed a two-hour ordeal in Spanish—I could never tell if I was the one suffering or the patient was, due to my Spanish skills—by performing a full history and physical exam on a seventy-four-year-old Hispanic woman. When I finished, she told me in perfectly plain English, "Your Spanish sucks, Doctor."

Lesson learned. Never assume, because it makes a you-know-what out of you and, well, just you, really.

Back then, we never rounded on all patients as a team; doctors were too busy. But there was some overlap for continuity of care so as to prevent disasters. Thus by design, the intern, resident, and attending never started the rotation on the same day. As a result, I would see some patients on my own.

Early on during the rotation, I wrote a daily progress note on the chart of a patient for three consecutive days and examined him every day independent of the team. On the fourth day, I told the patient, Mr. Jones, that he was going home because the carotid Doppler ultrasound of his neck to check for blockage of blood flow to the brain was normal.

He looked at me with a blank stare and stated, "I don't know what you're talking about."

To refresh his memory, I described the test where they put a jelly-like substance on his neck and listened for a "swoosh swoosh" sound to check for blockage. He looked dumbfounded, and once again told me that he had no idea what I was talking about. With growing frustration, my normal Michael Jackson tone had morphed into a full Bob Dylan scream. Despite that, he insisted he didn't know what I was talking about.

By now, I was annoyed, and told him I had the report in my pocket and showed it to him. *That's right Niraj, show him the evidence.* He politely told me he was not Mr. Jones.

Yes, you guessed it. I had rounded on the wrong patient and written on the wrong chart for the last four days. You're probably wondering if I'd spoken to this man during my bedside visits. Yes, I had, but not by name. Lesson learned: Always treat the patient by name, not by disease or alleged bed location. The real intern taking care of the patient was also writing daily progress notes on the same chart. There were so many damn notes on the chart that I'd never looked at the other intern's notes. Who had the time?

When I asked Mr. Not Jones why he had failed to inform me of my mistake, he simply told me that he had a side bet going with the other intern about how many days my buffoonery would continue. Frankly, he was angry because the over/under was seven days and he had placed his money on the over. He'd lost the bet.

The highlight of Harvard's rotation came towards the end of the month. It was the day after a busy call night, and I was presenting yet another patient with alcohol-induced liver cirrhosis, a form of chronic progressive liver failure that was commonly seen at The County. I presented the details of the history and physical exam. For privacy, these presentations were always delivered outside the patient's room, which at LBJ contained four patient beds artificially separated by thin curtains.

Harvard abruptly pulled the curtain and the bed sheet on my patient, turned to me and screamed. "My God, Niraj, you didn't tell me this man has an obvious case of leprosy!"

What are you talking about, Harvard? You have finally lost it, man, I said to myself. Since every intern's goal, including mine, was to somehow prove the attending wrong, I went straight to the library after rounds. *I'll show Harvard,* I said to myself. *Leprosy, my ass!* I didn't know much about leprosy that day, but I was sure my patient didn't have it.

I didn't sleep for the second consecutive night, and I came back to the hospital early the next morning to repeat the entire history and physical exam on the patient with alleged leprosy. On rounds the next day, Harvard made no mention of leprosy. Being brave or stupid, depending on your point of view—no one ever questioned an attending—I stated to

Harvard, "Sir, you mentioned yesterday that this man has leprosy and I missed it. Respectfully, I didn't go home or sleep last night. I came back and repeated the entire history and exam and respectfully, sir, I don't think this man has leprosy."

I thought my entire team was going to kill me. The attending would now make the rest of the month miserable for everyone because someone had had the nerve to question him. In fact, my inner voice was screaming, *What were you thinking, genius?*

Harvard turned to me, smiled, and responded. "Niraj, I know that, but aren't you glad you know so much more about leprosy now?"

Lesson learned. Lasting knowledge comes from an effort and motivation that is internal, and sometimes we need to determine how to maximize self-learning long after the attending is gone.

Fear no one, but always fear your own lack of knowledge.

14

Enemies

Arrogance kills.

Every medical student, and thus by extension every resident, knows this axiom early in their training: "Internal medicine and surgery don't get along." I am stating this in mild, respectful, non-vulgar terms. But this was quite true.

How else could you explain the jokes bouncing back and forth between the two departments?

"What do you call a double-blind study?"
"Two surgeons looking at an EKG."

"Why do surgeons use their heads to keep the elevator door from closing instead of their hands like everyone else?"
"Because they don't need to use their head in the Operating Room."

"Why do patients on medical services go home sooner than on surgical services?"
"Because the patients sign out against medical advice after one week of testing and the internist still doesn't know what is wrong with the patient."

"Who would a flying pig or a striped unicorn go to see if they got sick?"
"An internist because no one else would actually recognize their imaginary existence."

It was a tug-of-war between two services trying to one-up each other's micturition stream. Sadly, the patient was often stuck in the middle. I remember a case where the patient was admitted to the Medical Intensive Care Unit (MICU) team, with the diagnosis of sepsis. The MICU team and the surgical team's favorite word is *sepsis*. Everybody is septic and thus suffering from sepsis until proven otherwise, which was usually and often, though, proven or disproven only with an autopsy.

This particular patient was not doing well. I was a member of the MICU team, and we believed the patient had an intra-abdominal infection that was driving the impending multi-organ failure. Yes, this patient desperately needed to be taken to the Operating Room before he became even "more septic" (By "more septic," I meant, "before he died.") As such, the surgical team was consulted.

By now, God Wanna Be (GWB) from my medical school days had become Beyond God (BG). By simply touching the patient, he declared, "This patient does not have a problem with his belly requiring acute surgical intervention, but he is septic."

Huh? The MICU team, in full internal medicine mode, retorted, "Well, what the hell do you think is the cause of his sepsis?"

The answer actually came from me under my breath—or so I thought—at the same time BG spoke. "Because I've seen acute abdomen more than you have, and this isn't an acute abdomen. This is sepsis because this is what sepsis looks like! It's not coming from his belly."

I had heard this countless times during my surgical rotation. And BG said the exact same thing this time once again. Sadly, so did I.

BG looked me in the eye and made a statement I had also heard repeatedly during my surgery rotation. Until that day, however, I never had the courage to answer back. Unfortunately for him, he misspoke in the heat of battle. Usually, he would say "I'm better than you because my sphincter tone is tighter than yours" as if to imply some sort of toughness. Sponge Bob and I were similar in that we were both visual learners. Using your imagination, however, was not always a good thing.

On that day, he put his foot in his mouth by saying, "Remember what I taught you when you were a medical student? I'm better than you because my sphincter tone is higher than yours."

Having had enough of his nonsense, I responded, "I know! I know your sphincter is higher than mine because I can actually see it when you open your mouth, and that's why I see crap coming out of your mouth every time you open it!"

The entire medical team was on the floor rolling with laughter. The surgical team, including the medical students and interns, was snickering under their breath. BG looked at me, hoping to vaporize me with the intensity of his glare. Really, spontaneous combustion? *You are dumber than I thought,* I was thinking, as if I was also a mind reader. It was a dumb and dumber stare down.

When BG found me still standing there, he screamed, "I'll deal with you later, you shit!" Both upper-level residents of each service were now screaming at each other in spite of my impromptu humorous interlude. Nurses intervened, and attendings of both services amazingly materialized, which was a surprise to me. You see, on the MICU team, we only rounded with the fellow (attending junior) on most occasions.

As you know from the golf course days, most surgical attendings could only be found in the Operating Room (and golf course), not on the wards, especially not the internal medicine wards or MICU. I think surgical attendings viewed rounding as a form of punishment.

That day, true to form, both attendings sparred with one another, hurling political jabs back and forth. No conclusion was reached. Of course, the patient was septic, but no one agreed on why. Unfortunately, the patient eventually died, and the death certificate stated "sepsis" as the cause of death, just like it did for many other patients.

I was reminded of a quote by someone during my medical school that seemed harsh at the time, but struck a chord with me on this particular occasion. "Residents never learn from their mistakes because they bury them." Did this patient die of sepsis? Did he even have sepsis? We will never know, because an autopsy wasn't performed. His family had many questions, but we just gave them the usual sepsis speech.

Another lesson learned. I hoped that someday I could arrange a cease-fire in the turf wars between internists and surgeons, and therefore help the patient regardless of whether he or she had sepsis. Sadly, patients sometimes seem to die of a greater disease: the combined arrogance of the doctors taking care of them.

15

Solidarity

Attendings are pretendings.

With the daily drama between different specialties, exhausting working hours, and the general attitude of "I wish I was anywhere but here," how exactly were any of us learning? On the one hand, we had heard the Osler quote a million times about going to the sea without a boat and patients or some pithy wisdom like that, but I don't think Osler ever admitted twenty-seven patients in one day. (The actual quote was, "He who studies medicine without books sails an uncharted sea, but he who studies medicine without patients does not go to sea at all." But that wasn't much comfort at the time.)

We hoped to have an attending like Harvard from time to time, but only in small doses, because after a while we couldn't understand what he was saying. I remember a time when my resident asked Harvard how much Lasix (a diuretic medication used to remove excess fluid from the body) the patient should receive. Harvard replied, "I think this man has worked hard his whole life and this is just not fair!"

Now, you must remember that in the era in which I trained, shit pretty much rolled downhill and usually the intern—that would be me—was at the bottom of the hill. So we subconsciously were glad to see medical students on the service: someone else could be at the receiving end of the daily gravity-defined action.

Our training was like Lieutenant Dan in *Forest Gump* when he told the troops to "sit down and shut up." Just like in the movie, when the attending spoke, we heard the same phrase. And just like Forest replied in the movie, "so we did." No one spoke on rounds unless they were spoken to. I tried to follow this advice, but as you have probably learned by now, I wasn't very good at it.

The resident in charge of prescribing the correct dose of Lasix thus didn't ask the same question again. To do so would have been suicide, but it was obvious he was thinking, *What the hell are you talking about, Bowtie? Speak in English and remind yourself we're in the twentieth century.*

So, as usual my resident made the best estimation of how much Lasix he should give the patient. On the following day, the patient was still suffering from "volume overload" (too much fluid in the body) and needed more diuretic (Lasix). Harvard turned to my resident and asked how much Lasix the patient had received. The resident replied 40mg.

Harvard turned crimson red. "My God, man. What school of homeopathic medicine did you attend in India?"

"Here we go again," I said under my breath.

The resident was puzzled because although he was Indian like me, we both considered ourselves American, having grown up in the U.S. since childhood.

Harvard screamed louder as the resident continued to maintain his *Maun Vrat*. "I asked you a question. What the hell did I tell you on rounds yesterday? Didn't I tell you yesterday to give him at least 80mg of Lasix?"

As usual, my inner voice bubbled to the surface. "Well, actually, sir," I started, "you said this man has worked his whole life and this just isn't fair. (*Shut up, Niraj,* my inner voice kept saying, and from the look in the resident's eyes, I could tell he was wishing he was at a homeopathic medical school in India at this very moment.) To be fair, I wasn't able to find an association between your phrase and how much Lasix I should give him, so I guessed. It's not the resident's fault, but mine. I was also thinking about how maybe drying him out too much by giving him too much Lasix wasn't such a good thing since twenty-five percent of the cardiac output goes to the kidneys, and I didn't want him to go into renal failure. I was also thinking that he's already deaf and if we gave him too much Lasix, how would we know if he has ototoxicity."

Yes, I had DOTM, Diarrhea of The Mouth. Harvard continued the tongue lashing, but by now it all sounded like the muffled sounds of the person taking my drive through order at McDonald's: "Wok, wok, wok, blah, blah, blah." I couldn't understand anything, but it was probably just as well, because I didn't know that someone who had lived a good life should get at least 80mg of IV Lasix.

Harvard left rounds—probably short of breath from all the screaming—and I thought I was about to receive tongue lashing round # 2 from my resident. Instead he said, "Thanks man, for saving my ass. You didn't have to, but I'm glad you did.

"Remember that attendings are just pretendings. They will rant, rave, and leave. Your patients' care during your training will only be as good as your upper-level resident's abilities. For now it's me, but eventually it'll be you. Remember what I taught you that first day?"

"Yes, you told me to feel free to call you anytime, just consider it a sign of weakness," I responded. That was why we never called our residents during admissions or any other time unless the patient was dying. Fear comes in many forms.

"Well, let me tell you a secret. That is a rite of passage because I want to know who will speak up, take charge, take the blame when it was not their own, and give credit to others when they should keep it. My resident did the same thing to me when I was an intern. Today, Niraj, you've passed the test and earned the right to call me anytime."

I was almost in tears. Lesson learned. Although we needed our patients, as Osler suggested, my teachers during training would be my upper-level residents. I added a degree to his name that day and called him a PhD (Professional Homeopathic Doctor). And for a moment, it seemed as if there was no gravity, and although shit was all around me, at least it was temporarily on an even playing field, not rolling downhill.

16

Commandments

It's only mumbo/jumbo if it doesn't work.

The most important commodity an intern valued was time. Although every day was busy, no day was busier than the on-call day, which started at 7:00 a.m. and ended when I returned home the next day around 8:00 p.m. Yes, time was so important that every intern developed a list of superstitious behaviors and activities. We hoped that this would prevent the pager from going off on call day, signaling the next admission. I was no exception and had my own Ten Commandments (see next page).

Like other superstitious beliefs, I'm not sure how helpful any of the Ten Commandments were during training, but I'd like to believe they worked. Everyone in training had their own list, but I never met an attending who was actually superstitious.

That is, never until that one day during a General Medicine Ward month. During our intern year, we had no choice as to which rotations we would be assigned to during the year and thus our supervising attending physician. For this

INTERN YEAR COMMANDMENTS

1) Thou shall not take off your shoes or socks on call days. Is there an evidence-based research paper on a fungus among us when it comes to this particular theory?

2) Thou shall always wear your lucky scrubs. This was always one pair, and interns were not good at laundry. Like we actually had time to do laundry.

3) If lying down for a few minutes, thou shall always position the pager in the exact same location every single time. No exceptions. For me it was on my chest.

4) Thou shall always take one specific route to the emergency room for the first admission to prevent future admissions. For me, the route was the side stairs next to the cafeteria at LBJ. The Cullen stairs at Hermann.

5) Thou shall always eat the exact same food item on call day. I scarfed down nachos with extra cheese and jalapeños, because frankly, vegetarian options were too damn healthy for an intern in those days.

6) Thou shall always ask the emergency room if surgery had seen the patient first and if not, why not? In this case, punting was better than receiving.

7) Thou shall never wander around the hospital, especially the emergency room during shift change. Lonely intern meant automatic admission.

8) Thou shall never comb your hair on call. Someone might feel sympathetic if they looked at you and saw you rumpled.

9) Thou shall drink only black coffee because cream and sugar meant admissions. At the time, this commandment seemed hard to follow. Although now by habit and taste, I actually love black coffee.

10) NEVER EVER MENTION HOW MANY ADMISSIONS YOU HAVE. Especially if you thought you were kicking the previous team's butt because they had admitted twenty patients in twenty-four hours but your team was lucky enough to get only nineteen.

particular month, my attending was an MD-PhD. Like many others with dual degrees, he believed that he was smarter than everybody else. I called him Peacock because from day one, he had a swagger about him and always seemed to be strutting around. What was his superstition? On call days, he had a routine. He would enter the room and head straight for the window without uttering a word. He would open the window—probably a good thing since most interns believed in that lucky stinky scrub rule—that faced right above the emergency room on the ground floor and yell, "Team B is on call today! That's right, folks, Team B is on call today! C'mon down, everybody. Just c'mon in. We're waiting for you!"

Terror filled our Team B faces. *Go eat some nachos*, I was thinking. He did this shout-out every fourth day when we were on call, and believe it or not, it was working. We were consistently taking in fewer admissions than the other three teams.

Then a miracle happened. It was our last call day for the month, and as usual Peacock strutted into our room and did his thing. The team chuckled and settled in for the day, following our own Ten Commandments. We didn't realize that the bizzaro day was about to begin. (If Seinfeld had bizzaro world, we had bizarro day.)

My co-intern—I called her Ponytail for obvious reasons—and I kept looking at each other and our pagers on bizarro day. At noon, we had no admissions. Later, at 4:00 p.m., still no admissions! Even at 7:30 p.m. after the shift change in the ER, our pagers had not gone off.

Neither one of us would risk calling the resident or walking to the emergency room. So we paged each other to test the pager system. Our pagers beeped, so they were working.

Midnight passed. No admissions. Then 4:00 a.m. Still no admissions! Neither one of us could sleep, although I had my eyes closed, beeper on my chest, socks, shoes, and lucky scrubs all intact, already having had my black coffee and nachos with extra jalapeños.

Finally 7:00 a.m. the next morning arrived with no admissions! We'd just accomplished what had never been done at our residency program. We'd found the Holy Grail: We'd pitched a perfect game—a no-hitter, in fact.

The resident was dumbfounded the next morning. It was the first time I'd ever seen a resident at a loss for words. Peacock strolled in at 8:00 a.m. and asked the opening question: "How many did we get?"

The resident by now was deaf and mute.

"Zero, sir," I replied.

"Yes, sir, zero," my pony-tailed parrot replied.

"It actually works. It actually works. $#@#%$%Q," Peacock started babbling like a madman, and none of us could quite make out what he was saying or if it was in English.

Yes, we all had our small victories through superstitions that did nothing more than keep the mind busy. And for a moment, there was no fear, but my intern year was simply a hope and a dream that had come true. In that moment, the entire room was filled with nothing but smiling tears. We should have opened the window, and let the deluge pour down onto the Emergency Room. After all, sharing was all we had.

17

Stupidity

Laugh at yourself, stupid.

Small victories were short-lived during my intern year, and the constant grind was the norm. I was so exhausted that sometimes I had no idea what day it was. I still remember vividly two particular instances that served as a reflection of my daily haze from exhaustion.

The first occurrence was during my emergency room rotation at LBJ: twelve hours on and twelve hours off. We also flipped between days and nights: 7:00 a.m. to 7:00 p.m. became 7:00 p.m. to 7:00 a.m. with a day off between the switch. It was a brutal rotation requiring constant adrenalin kicks in the form of black coffee. There were always three interns working during any shift, each assigned to work in different parts of the emergency room.

It was a Saturday evening, and as usual, the interns arrived fifteen minutes before shift change at 6:45 p.m. There was only one problem. On this particular evening, strangely, four interns showed up for work. Long before software for smooth scheduling of rotations had been invented, our chief medical residents had mastered the template for the year with all rotations, vacations, and doctors in case of emergencies accounted for. They drank more coffee than we did and had to deal with our constant complaints—which is how I assumed they had gotten so good at making schedule templates.

No one was sick that particular evening. If someone had been ill, the number of interns working the shift would still have been the same. We would've seen an unfamiliar face, the back-up intern. By deduction, this could only mean one thing: one of the interns who didn't need to be there had actually shown up to work on his day off.

"It's Saturday, you morons. One of you schmucks is not supposed to be here! It's your day off, you idiot!" I said. Little did I realize that I was Dostoyevsky's prize pupil for the evening: I was the idiot who had shown up to work on his day off. What could be more humiliating than calling someone an idiot and then realizing that the mirror does not lie?

I took my foot out of the seemingly misplaced rectum on my face, and whimpered home. Yes, exhaustion does funny things to people, like showing up to work on your day off.

The second instance of exhaustion leading to acts of stupidity happened a mere two months later. I was on the MICU rotation at LBJ where call hours were different from the emergency room. The MICU call was every third night with three upper-level residents, each paired with an intern to take call for a twenty-four-hour shift. Although we would finish rounds by around 2:00 p.m. the following day, our work was not typically completed until 8:00 p.m. By the time we reached home, it was 9:00 p.m., and we had been awake for thirty-nine hours without sleep.

We would all fight as interns for the Friday call. Really, Friday night call, you might ask? Were we delirious? Couldn't we get a date? No, there was actually a method to our madness in this seemingly strange request. You see, the

MICU protocol was that unless you were on call, you didn't come in on weekends. So, if you were on call Friday, you weren't on call again until Monday. This meant that once you went home at 9:00 p.m. on Saturday, you got the entire day off on Sunday!

How did we decide on the winner for the Friday night call? Rock/paper/scissors of course! And due to much practice and defeat, I'd become damn good at the classic game from my days on other rotations. I was ready for the MICU and easily won the contest and thus the right to be on call that Friday night. I had a Sunday off! I would watch some Rockets, some Oilers—hell, I'd even watch soccer, I mean football, on the Spanish channel.

Yes, there was a smile on my face that carried into Saturday morning. I would have the entire Sunday off! If Dwayne "The Rock" Johnson could've seen me that day, he would've been impressed. And I'd won by being the rock in rock/paper/scissors—even better.

Nothing could piss me off that Saturday, not even leaving for home at 8:30 p.m. I went home and crashed. I must have fallen asleep by 9:30 p.m., dreaming about being an attending when I was awakened by a familiar sound. *Damn it, pager!* I quickly looked at the time: 7:20 a.m.

What the hell is going on? I said to myself. *I'm gonna kill whoever is paging me on my day off.* The number was familiar to me: 4491, the MICU.

"Somebody is going to have an early funeral!" I yelled into the phone.

"Where the hell are you?" came the voice from the other end of the phone line. It was the other intern. I called him Paper-Thin because I was Rock and I had just kicked his thin "paper" butt a couple days ago, knowing the third intern loved scissors that I manipulated to cut the paper.

"It's my day off, dumbass," I retorted.

"It's Monday morning, genius!" he fired back. "We are prerounding with the fellow, and you're late."

My world came to a standstill. I looked at the alarm clock again and looked at the date stamp on my beeper. They both confirmed that it was Monday morning. I had somehow slept forty-six hours straight! How was that possible? Was Rip Van Winkle Gujarati? *Shut up, voice*, I said to myself, but the words had already come out loud over the phone.

"What? Who you tellin' to shut up? You're late for rounds and you owe me." The phone went silent. On call again! Out the door I flew. No need to change. Lucky scrubs were already on since I hadn't changed clothes since I came home. Please don't ask about my undergarments.

On the way in to work, my disbelief turned to laughter. I wondered if an intern had ever shown up to work on his day off and accused others of being stupid by showing up to work on their day off. Perhaps this intern hit the "idiot double" and missed a day of his life because he slept in, this time accusing others of bothering him on his day off.

I hoped that someday no matter how distraught my interns became, I could share this story with them as an attending. Perhaps for a moment they too would be touched by laughing tears. After all, Rocks need moisture too.

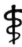

18

Stupid's Brother

FADOY over MADOY in a tight race

Intern year was full of stories. In the end, you hoped to not be immortalized as "The Story." By now, you're probably thinking that the award should easily be mine, and in fact should be renamed the MADOY (Mehta As Dumbass of the Year) Award. Sadly, I'd have agreed with you until I heard the story of Dr. Fingers, the name I gave him because he rescued me from becoming MADOY.

Dr. Fingers was on an emergency room rotation at a local cancer hospital in our program. As an intern, he was the front line troop member in sorting out potential but not obvious emergencies in cancer patients and subsequently presenting these cases to the upper-level resident. If the case was concerning, the resident in turn would consider presenting the information about the patient to the emergency room attending. The hierarchy was very important because of the high volume of patients; it was physically impossible for the attending of record to see every patient in detail.

During one of Dr. Fingers' shifts, a fifty-five-year-old woman with known cancer presented to the emergency room with nonspecific weakness. Dr. Fingers remembered that weakness in a cancer patient could be a manifestation of disease that has metastasized to the spine, and did an appropriate exam to make sure there was no spinal cord involvement. Although we were taught to look for a constellation of findings including weakness, hyperreflexia, a sensory level (meaning the patient felt a difference is sensation above and below a specific area on their body) and change in muscular tone, what we remembered the most was change in bowel or bladder function in a patient with spinal cord pathology. Since our physical exam skills were still at a rudimentary level and as such had problems with kappa values (a measure of inter-observer agreement) and reproducibility, we were taught to focus on the rectal exam, specifically the lack of rectal tone.

Dr. Fingers did the exam as usual and was not sure of the so-called "non-focal" neuro exam. In those days just like now, unless done by a neurologist, a non-focal neuro exam still means only one of two things: 1) I didn't do the exam 2) I did the exam, but might as well have not done it because I'm not sure of any of the findings. However, there was never a kappa value issue when it came to rectal tone—at least, we thought so until that day.

Apparently, Dr. Fingers felt no rectal tone on this woman with known cancer and was concerned about spinal cord involvement. In theory, there are stop-gaps to prevent the defecation from traveling seemingly against gravity. Murphy must have been in the emergency room that day and he must have laid bricks in his pants by the end of the shift. You see, the resident was busy in the shock room with one critically ill patient and the attending was busy in the other shock room with another patient. So Dr. Fingers had no one to confirm his findings.

He presented the case, and the resident asked Dr.

Fingers to order a STAT CT myelogram to assess for spinal cord involvement. In those days, this was no small task, even at a cancer center. A STAT study required significant concern by the ordering physician since the study itself would involve coordination of care involving multiple other players including the tech performing the study, the hierarchy structure within the radiology department, transportation, nursing, and finally the patient and their caregivers. At that time, there was no computer log-in from home, and therefore the radiology staff would have to come into the hospital to read the actual study. STAT was another way of saying "whoever ordered the study better be right because his or her butt is on the line for affecting so many other people."

In this case, no rectal tone meant STAT. The appropriate study was ordered, and as the lingo goes, the data was cooking. Dr. Fingers waited nervously, but was excited at the prospect of saving someone's life. Fortunately or unfortunately depending on one's point of view, the STAT CT was normal. If you've ever read any report by a radiologist whose favorite tree must be the hedge, a report is rarely if ever read as "normal." There are usually key words such as *mild, may, perhaps, clinical correlation recommended, or cannot rule out*. I think this was the radiologist's way of saying if I go to court, Jim Adler, the tough smart lawyer from Texas with commercials seemingly on every local late night channel at the time of my residency, isn't coming after me. Dr. Fingers' upper-level medicine resident was in shock.

"NORMAL? What do you mean NORMAL?! You guys never read anything as NORMAL," the internal medicine resident barked over the phone to the radiologist.

"Look, my staff is here and I'm telling you the study is completely normal," responded the radiology resident. He added, "Are you sure the neuro exam is abnormal, specifically there is no rectal tone?"

The internal medicine resident looked at Dr. Fingers, who responded, "I'm a hundred and ten percent sure."

Since his butt was also on the line, the internal medicine resident decided to perform his own neuro exam on the patient. He did not get any "nonspecific findings" like Dr. Fingers. Instead, he found a normal neuro exam. What about the rectal tone? The resident repeated the rectal exam, and the tone was. . . wait for it. . .normal.

For a second, the resident even entertained the thought (hopefully he wasn't a visual learner like me) about the differential diagnosis of transient or paroxysmal decrease in rectal tone. He quickly dismissed the idea, thank God, and arrived at one obvious conclusion: Dr. Fingers was in the wrong orifice near the rectum.

The resident turned crimson red, politely excused himself from the bedside, and asked Dr. Fingers to join him in the conference room. When the door shut to the conference room, he didn't know whether he should laugh, cry, scream, or all of the above. As it turned out, he did all three at once. I always knew upper-level residents were gifted compared to interns.

"You idiot!" he screamed at Dr. Fingers. "You were in her freaking vagina. I only have one more question for you. How many fingers did you use?"

I would have run out the door by now, but Dr. Fingers was still standing there. He sheepishly replied, "Three. That's why I thought it was real. I mean, I've never been able to get three fingers into a rectum before."

The patient was reassured and sent home. I can't say the same for Dr. Fingers.

Stories during residency—good, bad, or ugly—spread like wildfire and could make or break you. This was no exception. Over the next forty-eight hours, everyone knew about the STAT CT myelogram. I would have transferred out of the residency program, but not Dr. Fingers. He stayed and took a beating. In fact, for the next two years, whenever he was on call, he would receive random calls from other residents asking for a "STAT CT myelogram."

I know it sounds selfish, but then again, you would've been just as happy as I was when the world, at least temporarily, was cognizant not of MADOY (Mehta as Dumbass of the Year) but FADOY (Fingers as Dumbass of the Year.)

19

Closure

Mi Lopez no es su Lopez.

The intern year was coming to a close, and somehow I had survived. Or the patients had survived in spite of me, not because of me. Perhaps in retrospect, the patients kept coming back not due to the natural progression of their disease, but because we had made the wrong diagnosis. Or did we save them by accidentally making the right diagnosis? Maybe MD did stand for Mostly Dangerous. The story of Lopez from my intern year was the perfect illustration.

At LBJ, it wasn't uncommon to have a large number of Hispanic patients who didn't speak English. It was equally common for some of these patients to have the same last name. It seemed as if Murphy must have been my shadow during my intern year because once again I tried to recapture the MADOY from you know who. I was taking care of two patients both with the last name Lopez. One, Lopez 1, was admitted with a flare-up of his gout. The other, Lopez 2, was admitted with shortness of breath. I was asked to order a special test known as a ventilation-perfusion scan (V/Q) on Lopez 2 to make sure he did not have a pulmonary embolus—

a blood clot—in his lungs. Once again, there were no stop-gaps or electronic medical records to prevent mishaps.

There were four patients to a room at LBJ and the four charts were in little cubbyholes right next to each other by the door to the room. The label on the outside of the chart had the name *Lopez* and the location of the patient, including room and bed number. As luck would have it, Lopez 1 and Lopez 2 were in the same room, across from each other, and thus the charts were located right next to each other. I placed the order for the V/Q scan in the chart. The result came back a few hours later and was read as "high probability," suggesting that this was a medical emergency no matter how stable or comfortable the patient looked.

There was one problem. Well actually more than one, but let's start with the first. Our pretest probability or likelihood that Lopez 2 was having a blood clot in his lungs was low. Thus the study finding didn't match our clinical suspicion, narrowing the likely explanation to one of two scenarios: 1) Our likelihood was wrong, or 2) The findings of the study were wrong.

I presented the findings of the V/Q scan to the resident, who replied, "That's impossible." Having recently heard about Dr. Fingers' escapade at the cancer center, my inner voice spoke to me, *Be careful what you say. Anything is possible.*

"Why don't I go back and repeat the history and exam and get back to you in thirty minutes?" I suggested. The resident agreed and off I went.

After examining the patient, I was beaming ear to ear, still confident that the likelihood of a pulmonary embolus was low. Like a proud recruit, I presented my findings to the resident, and he for once agreed. What happened next? Well, in those days, every service wore a badge of pride and honor and went out of their way to let another service know that their service sucked or somehow had screwed up. This was no exception. Or so I thought. Yes, this disgrace was too good for a simple phone call.

"Let's go down to Radiology and tell that idiot to look at the V/Q scan again," said my resident. We were so excited to have an opportunity to prove somebody wrong. It was once again time to show Radiology that Internal Medicine was the boss. The radiology resident was well known to us. She was always right and had a condescending way of telling us we were wrong. Yes, baby, the tables were about to turn. Actually, we didn't know it yet, but they were about to turn on us.

My resident spoke, and I listened to my master, standing beside him like a faithful puppy. "You read the scan as high probability on Mr. Lopez, but we're confident that could not be the case. We're certain that the likelihood of this gentleman having a PE is low, and that means that you're wrong. Read the scan again, and frankly make an addendum to your report acknowledging your error,"

Wow, I thought to myself. *Can't wait to be an upper-level. And look, he said "we." I'm part of the "we." Yes, baby, I have arrived.*

Within the next five minutes however, I wished that somehow I could have departed without notice.

"Mr. Javier Lopez—" began the radiology resident, the smugness evident in her voice.

"You mean Francisco Lopez?" retorted my resident.

"No, I said Javier Lopez, and if I wanted to say Francisco Lopez, I would have said Francisco Lopez," she stated slowly, as if we were Dumb and Dumber.

Suddenly, Dr. Fingers came to mind, and served as a reminder that the differential diagnosis is always broader when an intern is left in charge of someone's care. Did I order the right test on the wrong patient? Impossible, how could someone be so stupid? Unfortunately, someone can, and that someone was me. The V/Q scan intended for Lopez 2 was ordered by genius me on Lopez 1. And it was positive. What the hell? We—I guess I should say I—weren't even considering a PE in a man admitted for a gout flare-up. I'm sure my resident was probably wondering if I was "relation" to Dr. Fingers, like Forrest and Bubba in *Forrest Gump*.

By now, the radiology resident (Smug, as I called her from that day forward) had figured out what had happened. Smug reminded us that the most important thing about a test is to order it on the right patient, although she was unaware of any papers about improving such probability and thus by extension patient outcomes. Smug continued that she would look for such papers, and that perhaps we could come up with a series of patients by next year for an observational trial.

We crawled out of the room, and I was reminded by my resident that I was Dumb and Dumber *(See, Mom and Dad, maybe I'm an Indian demigod with two personalities at once)*. Fortunately, Lopez 1 and Lopez 2 did fine. Yes, I went back and did another history and physical exam on Lopez 1 and discovered he was at risk for an asymptomatic blood clot.

Another lesson learned. *Two wrongs do make a right?* I thought to myself. *Mi Lopez no es su Lopez,* I quipped again, talking to myself as I entered House of the Lopezes.

"Your Spanish sucks, Señor," said Lopez 1 in his broken Spanglish. Lopez 2 burst out laughing. I started to laugh, too, and we all shared an impromptu moment of meaningful doctor-patient relationship.

With that, my intern year had come to a close. Although I had learned so much, I felt more confused than ever. I could tell, however, that I was slowly changing. I couldn't exactly put a finger on it, but somehow I was growing. It was hard to see at the time, but we were maturing into doctors who somehow made fun of our training and all of its shortcomings, but still cared about our patients. I wondered in the end if human beings, be it patients or doctors, had the same hopes and fears, and by extension, the same dreams and tears? Was I a doctor or a philosopher—or both or neither? Maybe I was just confused. Perhaps the second year of my residency would shed some light.

20

Signs Non-Zodiac, A Transition

DOSOTORAI becomes DOSOTORAIFUS.

The first six months of internship provided a steep learning curve in proficiency. The following motto summarizes the curve succinctly, although without much elegance. "Do one, screw one, teach one, read about it." We just called it DOSOTORAI. The latter half of internship provided the efficiency needed to match the proficiency since the mountain of patients to be taken care of was endless. The second-half motto? "DOSOTORAIFUS: do one, screw one, teach one, read about it faster U shit!" And you thought there were only twelve signs in the zodiac. Fueled by too much caffeine and not enough sleep, my mind would start to wander off at times, in search of answers to questions about the zodiac that should have been reserved for my psychiatric patients. I wondered more than once that if the patient came from the Age of Aquarius, would his outcome be dependent on whether his DOSOTORAIFUS was a Sagittarius? Alas, as you may have guessed, no funding for such research was available. Just in case someone asks, I'm a Virgo, so no virgin jokes, please. Some parts of the intern year are better left unsaid. Second year, ready or not, here I come...

21

Food For Thought

The Nazi cafeteria

Since I had mastered being a DOSOTORAIFUS, the first part
of the second year of residency actually provided previously
unheard-of time for observations. For starters, there was the
cafeteria. It was . . . how should I put this? Let me just come
out and say it: It was a Nazi regime, a dictatorship from top to
bottom. At least that was our perception. The cafeteria had a
strict policy for its hours of operation, and this policy, like all
other policies during my training, was non-negotiable. It was
not uncommon (since the mountain of patients that each one
of us was assigned was seemingly insurmountable) for most
residents, including myself, to eat just one meal a day. For a
vegetarian working his butt off at the county hospital, this
meant breakfast, but only from 6:30 a.m. to 9:00 a.m. NO
EXCEPTIONS! 6:29 a.m.? NO. Flying in the door at 9:01
a.m. after I just finished coding a patient? ABSOLUTELY
NOT! "Come back at lunch," said the cafeteria soldiers.
Never mind that the patient had just passed away, and seeing
his food tray at the bedside suddenly made me realize that I

had not eaten yet. Sad but true.

"What time would lunch be?" I asked the server, whom I had labeled Adolf in my mind. Saying *please* and arguing was a waste of time since my code beeper could go off at any time. But then again, I was having one of those days, and my patience was worn thin from an entire year of such BS.

"Read the sign on the door you came through," said Adolf.

"Why don't you just tell me since I'm standing in front of you?" I responded back.

"Read the sign on the door you came through,"

"I came in through the EXIT door. There is no sign there."

"You're not allowed to come in through the EXIT door. When you come back for lunch, come in through the ENTRANCE DOOR and read the sign."

"Will there be a separate sign for lunch hours or is it the same as breakfast hours?"

"It's the same, sir."

"So you mean the breakfast and lunch hours are the same? I'm so confused. Could you please help me understand?"

"You know exactly what I meant." Adolf had little sense of humor.

Now that I took a closer look, she did have a Hitler-esque mustache. *Wait, was this facial hirsutism? Did I need to consider other features of virilization? Please Niraj, shut up, not before breakfast or you'll throw up.*

"No actually, I have no idea. You see in my country, sometimes breakfast and lunch are all mixed up, and you know Indians like me, we just come here, for better life to help family back home." The awkward grammar and fake accent popped out.

"Sir, I don't like your tone," stated Adolph.

"What means you by that? This is criminal. You have word for this country—I mean in this country—for this thing this thing you do. RACISM. I will telephone and if busy I will write to NAABP. That's right, I will write, call collect, whatever it takes, you are RACISM, I mean you are racist!"

"Sir, calm down, lower your voice. People can hear you."

"You lower your voice and then I will lower mine and then in loud cafeteria and no one hears each other what you says about that, huh RACISM?!"

"Sir, I don't need your attitude, I'm just doing my job, I know people in the NAACP and there is no NAABP!"

"Ahh, see your tone now what you think about (*If it lateralizes to ear with hearing loss is that Weber or Rinne test positive or negative and is that conduction or sensory neuronal hearing loss? Shut up, Niraj!*) "And there is NAABP, I tell you. I know! I'm a carrying card member. It is Nationalistic Associations for Assisting Brown People (Yes, I really said that) and you big I mean trouble, I mean both." *Shut up, Niraj!* I be back lunch through the right door or left door or whatever and I will tell you what hours is lunch, breakfast, supper, dinner, snacks and yes whatever else. Have shitbull day. Good bye!"

For once, Adolf was speechless, her mouth wide open and eyeballs ready to pop out. *Was Munch German too? What is that cut off for exopthalmos for African American Woman? Please. For your own safety, shut up, Niraj.*

I chose to exit via the entrance door for my own twisted emotional closure and glanced back at her a few times, thinking, *Man, that mustache is growing fast. Adolf will look like Salvador Dali by the end of the day. Was she digoxin toxic?* I wondered, thinking about the half-Salvador Dali mustache resembling the sagging of ST-segments I was taught to look for on an EKG.

Everyone wondered why I was smiling the rest of that day and musing about Nazi regimens at The County. Just in case you were wondering, I did go back for lunch, coming in through the EXIT door, saluting the Führer on the way in and strutting out the ENTRANCE door.

22

Pretending

Everyone is in PP.

The interesting thing about starting the second year of residency is that no one was who they seemed to be. I was now leading the team as an upper-level resident, but only yesterday I was an intern! Yes, on June 23rd I was an intern, but on June 24th I became a resident! In fact, during my training, there were unconfirmed rumors circulating about lawyers settling litigation between June 24th and July 31st at all hospitals that had academic affiliations (i.e., institutions where residents were taking care of patients). This made sense since it was technically the first month of training, and everyone was essentially playing a part they hadn't memorized the script for yet.

Yes, your memory is correct. I was sued as a medical student during the same time frame, and yes again to your question about the settlement. I called this first month transition the Poser Period, or by its unfortunate abbreviation PP for short. The crazy thing: I wasn't PPing alone. At times, the attendings were residents the day before, and wanted to explore the academia lifestyle for a year or two. I think they were just scared to throw themselves into the real world of private practice. Consult fellows who were supposed to be experts in their field were on day one of their fellowship and thus also wet behind their ears. Interns were medical students the day before, and given the rampant senioritis in medical school (remember my golf rotation), most hadn't seen a patient in at least a month, if not longer. The medical students were actually in classrooms the day before, and were eternally confused.

No one told the patients to be patient during PP, although the number of readmissions during the transition period was always the highest. Coincidence? I think not. In fact, patients during PP had to have nine lives to survive in spite of us, not because of us. No, I never said that out loud— to a patient, that is.

23

I Am In Charge

Shit rolls downhill both visibly and invisibly.

PPing was everywhere, which leads me to my welcoming speech for the team. After all, I was now the top dog. We called attendings "pretendings" because they had all the theory but no practicality. Or was it all practicality but no theory? Unbeknownst to me at the time, someone in Canada had already coined the term "evidence-based medicine" to combat such a dilemma. Alas, we were in Canada South (or was it Mexico North?) for now.

Oh, how I missed Harvard (the attending, not the school that refused to accept me even in my dreams). But, I digress, so let's get back to my welcoming speech for the team. I had heard so many versions of the "Friends, nobleman, countrymen, lend me your ears" stuff since my medical student days that I was a bit overwhelmed with the possible choices. Which style should I pick? Military, Mother Teresa, Mr. Rogers (for you youngsters: Google that PBS reference), or something else? Should the tone be firm, as was the norm in my surgical rotations, or gentle like my psychiatric rotations? It seemed as if I had AMC 26 movie theatres playing famous lines in my head….

Remember, your patients are like the *Terminator*: *"They'll be back."*

From the famous Forrest Gump: "Call is like a box of chocolates*; you never know what you're gonna get."* Privately though, that's how upper-level residents felt about new interns as well as pretendings.

From *Ferris Bueller's Day Off*: *"Life moves around pretty fast and no you don't have time to sit around. Yes, for the next three years, you are gonna miss it."*

From *Lethal Weapon*: *"I'm too old for this shit"*

From *Wall Street: "Lunch is for wimps."*

From *Poltergeist*: *"They're here."* The patients, that is.

From *Ghostbusters*: *"Human sacrifice, internists and surgeons working together, mass hysteria!"*

From *Sudden Impact: "Go ahead, make my day."*

From *A Few Good Men*: *"You won't get answers, you are not entitled to the truth, and no, you can't handle the truth."*

It seemed as if residency was just one never-ending movie where the same crap happened over and over again. Was *Groundhog Day* filmed at LBJ?

After what seemed like an eternity of deliberation, I settled on the "picture is worth a thousand words" approach. I drew stick figures in a vertical plane with the most menacing at the top. The figures became smaller and less threatening. At the bottom was the gentle soul with pigtails and a dress or one with a pocket protector and *Revenge of the Nerds* glasses. In between each of these stick figures were some droplets/pallets.

I asked the new team what they saw. As usual, no one spoke. I asked about the differential of mutism and again there was silence. So, I started my simple explanation. "You see, the menacing guy at the top is me, the resident, the leader, the badass, the savior, and the greatest. I'm in charge and I don't like getting crapped upon. But sometimes there are invisible forces that are crapping on me. Yes, you are correct—you don't see them because well they're invisible. When they crap on me, they follow the principle of gravity. Shit rolls downhill, and these pellets are me crapping on you. Notice that you're on the bottom, and the pellets get smaller and smaller, and so do the stick figures."

I stopped talking and looked at them. Still they remained silent.

"Yes, you don't need to know the Krebs Cycle anymore, but you need to know the Crap Cycle, and I shit bigger than you. Does anyone know what movie this is from?"

Silence again.

"*City Slickers*, damn it! What did you do for four years in medical school or college?"

Still there was pin-drop silence, which was extremely rare at The County. They were starting to look like lambs and I was starting to feel like Hannibal Lecter, even though I'm a vegetarian.

"So, in conclusion, don't try to defy gravity and you'll be fine. By rounds tomorrow, know twenty causes of mutism. Any questions?"

Finally, a brave soul raised his hand. "Hum, Dr. Mehta, I was, hum, wondering where is the attending on your picture?"

"Excellent question," I retorted. "He or she along with the surgeons and the ER make up the invisible forces that are constantly crapping on me. That's why they're not on the board, but they're real and very important."

The group shuffled out of the room and I smiled at myself. Or did I? I went back to the call room that day and didn't like the reflection I saw. Why was I trying to become someone I wasn't? This wasn't the guy I started out as. Why did my tone have to be so harsh? It seemed as if everyone was bipolar in residency. You almost needed that mentality to survive the hours, the physical and mental anguish, and the loneliness that followed you like a shadow that never left, even in darkness.

But I didn't want to survive. I wanted to change. I guess I'd need to start with changing myself. I continued to struggle with this process well beyond residency, but at least this moment was the beginning of self-reflection and growth. I hoped to change one life at a time starting with my own. I dreamed that someday I would mellow, and learners below me would understand me. But I feared that all this would be for naught. I cried a tear, but there was no hand to wipe it. *Loneliness is such a cruel friend,* I thought.

I fell asleep until the beeper went off twenty minutes later. Wow, twenty minutes of sleep on a call day—a new record! *Was this on the board downstairs for the medical Olympics?* I wondered as I ran out of the call room down to my home within a home, also known as the ER.

24

Ward Call

The art of being The Wall

What a perfect segue as to what exactly defined a call night. Since I trained well before the Accreditation Council for Graduate Medical Education (ACGME) and Residency Review Committee (RRC) instituted the eighty-hours-per-week guidelines in 2003, my memories of call are quite different from those of current doctors in training. When I trained, it was especially brutal for the upper-level resident. To fully grasp the Herculean task that we faced, you must first understand and appreciate the call system at LBJ. We were on call every fourth day from 7:00 a.m. to 7:00 a.m. the next day. The team consisted of the pretending (unless it was Harvard), an upper-level resident (tragically during the PP, this was me), two interns (again glorified medical students during PP), and of course the medical students (regardless of PP or not, they were just dazed and confused).

There was no cap—no maximum ceiling on the number of patients that could be admitted to the team on call. What if there were no beds available? Well, the patients were still admitted to us. We simply cared for them in the holding area of the emergency room until a bed became available. Did we not have JCAHO, the national organization which certifies hospitals as meeting or not meeting the national standards of care, back then? Would it have made a difference? It seems that every time a hospital meets the standard of care, JCAHO changes the rules of engagement. How many times did I take a history and examine a half-clothed patient in the hallway? It was not unusual for patients to wait for up to forty-eight hours for beds. As the patient sat waiting, the holding area became increasingly crowded. After all, you couldn't lock the emergency room and prevent more patients from coming into the hospital.

Or could you? Ah, the beauty of the "drive-by." An unfortunate term since it brought back memories of drive-by shootings on my trauma rotation, but a blessed term nonetheless. If the emergency room attending, with approval from the hospital administrator, felt that every nook and cranny of the hospital was full, especially the emergency room, then the hospital was on "drive-by." All ambulances were told not to bring patients to drive-by hospitals unless the patient's condition was deemed unstable and emergency care elsewhere was not available.

Every time we would hear sirens, our collective heart rate would rise, but would slow down again as the sound faded. We were relieved to know that the ambulance had passed LBJ and was on its way to the next hospital. Since our hospital was located near the freeway, we would often stand on the back lot of LBJ and say to the passing ambulance: "Bye-bye, we're on drive-by!"

I've often wondered how many lives we actually saved this way. Don't get me wrong: We did provide care, but the number of patients requiring medical attention was endless, and we had limited time and resources—always a tragic and often lethal combination. On average, we cared for twelve to fourteen patients on our service heading into the twenty-four-hour call day. We also admitted up to twenty new patients from the emergency room on the call day. Using simple math, we were in essence responsible for one new admission every ninety minutes—in addition to providing care for the other patients already on the service. This was *Mission Impossible* long before the Tom Cruise movie, but we had a system that made survival possible.

How did we survive and what was our system? It was a game called "The Great Wall of China," or "The Wall" for short. The goal of the upper-level resident was to block every admission to his or her service. I wasn't the only one playing the game: every single upper-level resident played, and some were better at it than others. Worse, this game wasn't restricted to the medicine service. It was played on *every* service.

My motto was "you are too sick or too healthy to be on my service." If you were too sick, you needed to be admitted to the Medical Intensive Care Unit rather than my team. Of course, when I was on the MICU service, the motto changed a bit: "You're too healthy to be admitted to my MICU, and I don't have enough beds. What limited number of beds I have available, I must protect for the next patient who may come in at any minute and require a ventilator. Wait, I hear a siren. That could be it!"

You had to be careful, though, because all residents in the internal medicine training program would rotate through every service. Eventually, they would be in charge of the ER, the MICU, or the hospital team. If you burned your bridges with colleagues, well, life would indeed be miserable for you. In the end, the particular training specialties stuck together, just like they did during medical school. It was basically one fraternity thinking they were going to one-up the other and be The Wall. Thus, residents training in one department tried to transfer patients to all other departments.

Psychiatry did not have an inpatient unit at LBJ, but there was always an Axis II medical problem driving some patient crazy. I don't think a naked patient running around in the emergency room saying "I am Jesus, I am Jesus" needed medical clearance before being transferred to an inpatient psychiatric facility. This was especially true when we were seeing the patient for the twentieth time this year. I think his "routine labs" that had been normal for nineteen consecutive admissions would . . . uh, let's see . . . once again be normal! I think we were just annoyed because Psychiatry had mastered being The Wall, and there wasn't a damn thing we could do about it.

So, like a ping pong ball, the patient's potential admission would bounce back and forth between multiple upper-level residents. Now that I think about it, each one was thinking "I am God," not too different from the aforementioned psych patient. *Wait, Jesus was the son of God. Never mind.* This is what happens with one's convoluted thought process during training. At times, there were more "Gods" on call at LBJ than there were in India. *(Don't be mad, Mom and Dad. It was true.)*

Indeed, a ping-pong diplomacy—or lack thereof—was at play. The ER would try to admit a patient with a diabetic foot ulcer and uncontrolled hypertension to me to "rule out osteomyelitis," an infection of the underlying bone. I would respond, "He has a psychiatric problem and that's why he doesn't take his damn meds! Besides, he is a frequent flyer (someone who comes to the hospital often) and this has been ongoing for six months. Why does he need to be admitted now? Did you call the surgeons already?"

I knew the answer, but it was still worth a try. Yes, Surgery God said, "Thank you for this interesting consult, but the patient is not an ideal surgical candidate. I would admit to Medicine for IV antibiotics and further risk modification. A surgical procedure may be deemed appropriate in the near future after the patient's nutritional needs have been appropriately addressed."

"He is homeless, ER God, can't you see that! How am I going to fix his nutritional needs? He probably eats more than I do during this goddamn residency!"

"Calm Down, Medicine God. I too was a Medicine God a couple of months ago. This God is on your side, but I can't do anything. My hands are tied."

"Did you talk to ER Super God?" I asked the ER God.

"Yes," he replied. "It took me an hour to find him, but he told me to figure it out on my own. I also asked the Surgery Super God to put a note on the chart and his addendum to the Surgery God note reads: 'Agree with above.'"

"Damn it! I'm Admitting Medicine God. Between you and me, we don't like the MICU Admitting God. Can't we just send the patient to him and deem it safer for the patient to be in a more controlled environment?" I asked the ER God, my voice now sounding like the Bollywood actor I had seen play the role of Krishna as a child.

ER God told me he that was on my side and retorted, "I tried, but Bastard, I mean MICU Admitting God says he is only taking patients that are sicker than sick. Bastard told me don't call him unless the patient has been coded a couple of times in my ER, already intubated, and I can't admit him to the Surgical God. Sick bastard that MICU Admitting God!"

"Fine, I'm sending my Admitting Dumbass Intern down to talk to your Dumbass Intern."

"Thanks Admitting Medicine God," said the Emergency Room God. "Remember when we were dumbass?" he asks.

After a brief pause I reply, "We still are. Just don't let anybody find out."

So, that is how a typical call night went. Everyone was completely exhausted from lack of sleep and trying to be The Wall. You might think our energy would have been better spent just accepting new patients. Not true. It's hard to explain, but ask a doctor in training what he or she would give to have even two fewer admissions per call, and you'll understand our thought process. Although humorous and tragic at the same time, the sheer volume of patients and limited resources made us very efficient. We had no choice. Survive, or go home and be laughed at as the one who quit. We didn't have hours to consider things, nor did we have apps to instantly spit out answers.

As Osler suggested, our patients became our books, and all of us in training became each other's consultants, recognizing our strengths and weaknesses. We took care of the sickest. Along the way, we learned which patient really didn't need to be admitted, even if we decided so for the wrong reasons. I used to wonder if one of those gods from LBJ or some other similar training program actually went to the dark side and became an insurance company CFO or hospital administrator. After all, don't gods have the same hopes and fears and dreams and tears as those beneath them? Sadly, not yet…

25

Morning Report

Welcome to non-negotiable.

After trying to be a model of proficiency and efficiency while multitasking as The Wall on overnight call, what could be worse? Morning report.

At 7:00 a.m. sharp, the residents from the four medicine teams would meet with a legend. I called him Dr. NN because he had strict rules and everything was *non-negotiable.*

At morning report, the two residents from the overnight team would present patients to Dr. NN. Since call had started the previous morning at 7:00 a.m., we were presenting without having slept for about twenty-four hours. Since we were completely exhausted, it didn't take much to be on the receiving end of a butt-kicking. "May I have another, sir?" became our motto.

Did I mention the rules for morning report? Here are the Ten Commandments I remember well (see next page).

We had heard many crazy stories about Dr. NN during our intern year. We could never confirm their veracity because interns weren't considered smart enough to attend his morning report. Residents always received an instant jolt of

MORNING REPORT COMMANDMENTS

1) Thou shall not be late.

2) Thou shall look at blood smears and urinalyses of relevance before presentation.

3) Thou shall know the admission chest x-ray on every patient.

4) Thou shall get medical records overnight regardless of where the records may be located.

5) Thou shall not interrupt morning report with your pagers/beepers going off.

6) Thou shall be excused from morning report if you are dead and have evidence to back up your claim.

7) Thou shall be responsible for all of your actions and will be accountable for those actions.

8) Thou shall not leave once you enter, even for bathroom emergencies.

9) Thou shall know the CARD.

10) Thou shall know that God's initials are NN and getting out of hell is, well...*non-negotiable*.

happiness by making interns pee their pants by exaggerating stories. Were these stories truly exaggerations?

Dr. NN was a profanity machine and would make Sam Kinison look like Mr. Rogers. I was told that we would go in thinking we knew what was wrong with our patient only to leave as babbling idiots. Legend had it that everyone would get a lump in the throat, be at a loss for words, and probably cry before the end of the month. In fact, rumors were so rampant that the third-year residents made bets about who would cry first.

The concept of morning report with Dr. NN reminded me of *The Shawshank Redemption* and "fresh fish" when the new prisoners arrived. Third-year residents warned us to stay awake and pay attention because flying objects were moving faster and were closer than they appeared. Yes, things were literally thrown during morning report. I was told that trying to defend yourself meant you had better know your stuff inside and out because Dr. NN had had his first morning report in 1956.

How old was this guy? I was told that he was an ultra-marathon runner. He apparently held records for running one hundred miles in the fifty-to-sixty-year-old division. *Is that miles per lifetime?* I wondered. He supposedly had written books and published so many clinical papers that for my safety, I was reminded to know in detail everything he had written. However, he didn't like "kiss ass" residents and could see right through them. In fact, he once asked how long there was shit on someone's nose because they had been…well…

You might be wondering if anyone had anything positive to say about Dr. NN. After all, he had been called many other colorful names that I'm sure would have been top entries in the Urban Dictionary had it been available in 1994. The administration had apparently tried to fire him but he had survived because, in spite of all his thorns, by the time residents finished their training, they worshipped him and lived by his commandments. In fact, many of his former residents were now supposedly chairmen of departments across the country.

Maybe he was God? But how could God be so mean? How could God scream all the time? How could God make me feel small and make me cry? And how could God have such a potty mouth? Over the next two years, I would have to make up my own mind. And like many other educators I encountered during my training, as you shall see, there was no middle ground. I would either love him or I would want to kill him. As it turned out, I…

The morning report room was located on the ground floor at LBJ, next to the radiology file room. I didn't realize it at the time, but the location of the room was critical. It was right next to the ER, making access simple after a night of call, since there were months I never saw the call room—or got any rest.

The ER entrance was the preferred mode of entrance for the two overnight or on-call residents. The other six residents, who were driving in from home, parked in the back lot. They would take the long hallway opposite the cafeteria. The morning report room was the last door on the right. A normal walk took twenty-seven seconds. A brisk walk took about twenty seconds. A mad dash that Usain Bolt would have been proud of: exactly five seconds. We knew the exact times because of one of the Ten Commandments: "Thou shall not be late." In NN's mind, 6:30 meant 6:30:00, not 6:30:01. In fact during orientation, our watches were synchronized to the clock in the morning report room, which had a second hand for precision.

The location next to the file room was critical since the file room contained the one piece of information that Dr. NN required on all of our patients: the chest x-ray. If we thought Dr. NN was non-negotiable, the workers in the file room were BNN, *Beyond Non-Negotiable.*

26

The Chest X-Ray

Welcome to another dictator from the Axis of Evil.

We were required to obtain a routine chest x-ray on all new admissions. Of course, we were given the opportunity to not order the chest x-ray if we felt it was not indicated. Really, not indicated? Imagine what Dr. NN would do to you in front of seven other residents if you were wrong. No thanks. Everyone was getting a chest x-ray, at least when I was a second-year resident. Dr. NN believed the chest x-ray would give him an idea of what was going on with the patient's heart, lungs, bones, upper abdomen, and other mediastinal structures in a cost-effective manner. This would obviate the need to actually see the patient, which would be impossible anyways in a morning report that was scheduled to be one hour long.

The problem: we didn't have EPIC/PAX or any other system of electronic medical record or imaging services. So the radiology file room was where we went to die before we would die all over again next door in the morning report conference room. I think I survived only because I was a Hindu and the birth/death cycle would lead to my reincarnation. That's what I kept telling myself, hoping it would not be a cycle that would repeat itself at LBJ—although during residency, it invariably did every fourth day of call.

You earlier met the fascist regime of the cafeteria. The theme of dictatorship seemed to exist in areas beyond the LBJ cafeteria. Adolf may have worked in the cafeteria but Mussolini appeared to be alive and well, working in the radiology file room. We had to check out all x-rays by submitting the patient's medical record number and the physical location of the patient on a small sheet of paper along with our pager number, full name, name of our team, and name of our department.

We took admissions until 6:00 a.m. Yes, I know technically until 7:00 a.m., but there was an unwritten rule in the emergency room: Medicine residents were about to get their butts kicked by Dr. NN. As a result, the ER would slow down the work-up on patients and order some nonspecific labs to delay admitting the patient until the next team arrived at 7:00 a.m. There were many days when I was that next team and had six admissions already waiting for me. Really?

But then again, we knew well before Justin Timberlake that "what goes around always makes its way back around," so we just took our licks, knowing the favor would be returned when we were finishing overnight call.

The problem with Mussolini was twofold. The first problem was that I was so busy that I tried to ensure that films would be ready by 6:30 a.m. for the 7:00 a.m. morning report. Most requests were made as I admitted the patient. So, I could have an 8:30 a.m. admission, nearly twenty-two hours before morning report, but I would still submit the request for the chest x-ray. This was ideal because it allowed me adequate time to view the film.

Well, I think Mussolini had a brother named Murphy who had his own law in the radiology file room. Just because you turned in the reservation for the chest x-ray didn't mean that somehow the film and/or the reservation would not be lost. *That's right, Jerry Seinfeld. Anybody can take the reservation, but the most important part of the reservation is to keep the reservation.* I used this line as well as other Seinfeldisms during training to keep my sanity. Unfortunately, Mussolini was not from NYC and didn't watch *Seinfeld*, not even the Soup Nazi episode.

The second problem with the Mussolini regime was that submitting requests in a timely manner was non-negotiable. However, some x-rays were done in the emergency room, and the process was more complicated. First, the cassette that had the x-ray would need to be taken to the processing room for development. From there, another worker had to transport the film to the file room. Finally, yet another worker was responsible for placing the x-ray in the correct patient's folder. With such a complicated process, there were no guarantees of having an x-ray ready for checkout even if the reservation was turned in on time. Breakdowns were common, and films could not often be found, leading to frequent butt-kickings.

Well, the butt-kicking was going to occur anyway, but perhaps this would be a kinder, gentler butt-kicking. NOT. The combination of late admission, portable films, and Mussolinis about to finish their shifts wasn't good for anyone. My stomach lining took the brunt of the beating, and was already on fire from four cups of coffee and six cans of Diet Coke, which constituted my daily stress diet.

Mussolini had the entire family working in the file room—everyone there looked like the Italian mafia. The conversations were the same and the results were the same.

"Hi, I turned in requests for the sixteen chest x-rays I need to check out this morning."

"When did you turn them in?"

"Well, throughout the day because I know how busy and overwhelmed you are," I would reply (*if you believe it, Niraj, it isn't a lie*).

"Don't get sassy with your tone."

"Huh? What tone? I mean, oh I'm sorry I didn't mean to upset you. I'm so sorry. It's just been a very busy night."

"That's not my problem."

"Yes, yes, I understand." That's when I'd look frantically at my watch. "Do you have the films, please?"

"Yes, here you go."

Count Niraj, count. 1, 2, 3... "Umm, excuse me. There are only fifteen films here, and I turned in sixteen reservation slips."

"I only see fifteen. Did you turn them all in to me?"

"No, well, because you weren't here."

"Well, they only gave me fifteen so that's why you get fifteen. Fifteen reservations mean fifteen films."

No matter how much I argued, I wouldn't get that sixteenth film. So just like that, I walked out with fifteen films for sixteen patients, preparing myself to say, "May I have another, sir?"

What was the second problem with the file room? If they couldn't hold reservations submitted well in advance of morning report, what do you think happened when the 5:30 a.m. ER admission came in? What were my chances of success if I walked in asking for films without a reservation? Did I mention that it was not uncommon for other services, including our sworn enemies the surgeons, to also need the same films? Whose reservation took priority, and why didn't somebody return the films from the day before? After all, reservations were only good for twenty-four hours. Did I mention that for Dr. NN, the most important thing for a current admission was to compare data points from the previous admission, and that the chest x-ray played an important role in this comparison?

And this chaos was just the appetizer for the main course. I wasn't very religious, but I prayed deeply every morning between 6:00 a.m., when I went to pick up the x-rays, and 6:59:59 a.m. before the slaughter began.

27

7:00:00 a.m.

The card that made you or killed you

The chairs in morning report were placed in a circle. Dr. NN sat strategically with a perfect view of the door. He was flanked by the chief medial resident, usually a politically correct, bright resident who was a yes-man and probably in need of a letter of recommendation for a fellowship. Dr. NN had a direct view of the clock. The two resident presenters sat directly across from Dr. NN right next to each other, perhaps to provide moral support. I think it was so Dr. NN could visualize which lamb he was going to eat first. The remaining residents took random seats, but usually the third-year residents sat next to each other. Yes, the formation was *Kumbaya*, but what was about to take place was anything but.

The format was set, and like everything else, it was—wait for it—non-negotiable. The key was the card, which Dr. NN had taken a lifetime to develop. Although I wondered, I was not about to ask him if he started his life's work as a baby.

As he had told us during orientation, he wanted to separate the "shit from the shinola" and didn't have time for our BS. He was proud of his favorite present, a roll of toilet paper given to him by previous residents, who inscribed a thank you on it for teaching them how to discern shit from shinola.

To save himself grief, he developed the card. For each new patient that was admitted to the team, a resident would turn in a 5x7 index card with the following information:

Name of Patient and Medical Record Number
Room/Location of patient
Patient's doctor if he/she had one prior to admission
Patient's Problem
Patient's Diagnosis

On the bottom of the card would be the signature of the resident. There would be no abbreviations on the card. This was important because the resident was responsible for this patient and would be held accountable—not the intern, not the medical student (usually that was a good thing), and certainly not the emergency room or the team attending. Did I mention that the problem and diagnosis had to be five words or less? Shit from shinola, remember.

The basic idea was that the patient's problem must remain the same, although the diagnosis could change as more data was obtained. It was also important to note that with rare exceptions, the symptom was not the problem. For example, the novice would think the patient's problem was shortness of breath and this would have a massive differential diagnosis involving multiple organ systems including the heart, lungs, brainstem, abdomen, or kidneys, not to mention hysteria. Dr. NN's approach was to narrow it down to an organ system, or what we would initially think was the disease and make that into the problem. Confused? Dazed and Confused? Most of us were both for the next few years and even after residency finished, but Dr. NN would be proud because the light bulb eventually went on.

For example, the problem would be congestive heart failure exacerbation, and the diagnosis would be atherosclerotic coronary artery disease. As Dr. NN read the card, we knew what was coming. Usually, his rules were not followed. "God damn, you lazy bastards, why can't you follow directions? Did you forget to take your freakin' IV Synthroid this morning or were you born with congenital myxedema so you can just blame it on mommy and pappy?"

These meetings were sarcastic and quietly entertaining if you weren't one of the two lambs on the menu? Most people with money went to dinner and a show. We went to breakfast and a show. Breakfast was a cup of coffee. And the entertainment was Dr. NN. Now that I think about it, it brings a tear to my eyes. What can I say? I'm nostalgic. At least now, the tears represent joy.

During the presentation, if somehow Dr. NN read the entire card—meaning your handwriting was legible, you used fewer than five words to describe a problem or diagnosis, you did not use any abbreviations, and you signed the card with handwriting that was again readable—then the question that followed was always the same: "What is your evidence?"

Dr. NN taught by the Socratic method of asking questions, and he was one of the few teachers who challenged me to think. Most residents, including myself, would start with, "The patient is a forty-seven-year-old male…"

"Is he a male kangaroo?" would come the reply.

This actually happened to me. I responded with silence.

"I asked you a question. Is he a male kangaroo? Is he from Australia? What airline did he come on? You can hear me, why don't you answer me?" He would turn to the other residents and ask them if they could hear him. Then he would turn back to me and repeat the question. "So, is he a male kangaroo?"

I finally answered, "No!"

"Are you sure?" he asked.

"Yes, I think so, I mean I'm positive." *Never let him see you sweat, Niraj. He is coming in for the kill. Doesn't he know that vegetarians don't taste as good?*

"Speak up. I can't hear you" he retorted.

"Yes, sir. I'm positive."

"Do you understand why we're spending so much time on what seems to you to be such a trivial point? Your patient is human and thus he is a man, not a male which is nonspecific related to species. I'm trying to clean up your damn language!"

"Sorry, sir."

"Don't apologize, just think before you speak. My question is what is your evidence for congestive heart failure?"

"Well, he sir is a forty-seven-year-old gentleman," I started. That was the end of attempt number two.

"What makes him a gentleman?" Dr. NN retorted.

"Excuse me sir, I don't understand."

"You just met him, so you don't really know him. How do you know he's a gentleman?"

"Well, I guess I don't."

"First of all, don't guess, and think about the term gentleman and what it means and implies. You can't assume things about people without evidence. Stay objective, stay focused, think much, and speak little. Now let's try this again before you continue to get my blood pressure higher and I collapse right here and probably die since I would have to be admitted to your goddamn team!"

I had had enough by now so now it was my turn. "Well, actually sir, it would be the next team since my call is over."

"Lucky for those patients going to the next team instead of you," he replied. "Which reminds me now that you have me distracted with your damn presentation, let's ask your colleagues. Does anyone know why God has given Mehta two rectums? Anyone? C'mon. We're here to learn and broaden our knowledge. Don't be shy. Anyone? Why has God unfortunately given Mehta two rectums?"

I was looking at my colleagues and my eyes were only saying one thing: *I don't care what year I am. I may be junior and smaller than you, but if you open your mouth to even consider answering this question, I will make your life a living hell!*

Luckily no one answered. Dr. NN chimed in. "It's because he has so much shit to share with the world that he needed two openings and so God blessed him with one here and another one here." He pointed to his mouth and his butt.

Breakfast and a show, remember? I was having chest pain and starting to wonder in my own mind what Killip class I would be when I had a massive heart attack right here in this room. And yet, people worshipped this guy! *I'll show him who I am. Just give me time.*

So, the torture continued, and I was brought back to reality. "So we know your patient isn't a kangaroo and you don't know if he is a gentleman or not. This leads me back to my original question per your card. What is your evidence for congestive heart failure?"

By now, I was tired and angry but somehow more focused. Maybe his method was working. "I heard an S3 on exam," I answered.

"Finally something comes out of one of your dual rectums that makes sense," he answered.

I was about to smile until the rectum analogy made me pucker up in more ways than one. I was in my deaf mode (answering before hearing) when the next question popped up

"How do you know what you heard is an S3?"

"Because it sounded like an S3?" I responded, now completely confused, wishing I was in the mute mode instead.

"How does an S3 sound? Tap it on the wall."

I tapped on the wall using my knuckles to generate three heart sounds.

"Interesting," he responded. "What else sounds like an S3 in early part of diastole?" he asked.

I was silent. Another resident softly spoke, "An opening snap, Dr. NN."

"Excellent. Now we're having a discussion."

Thus the Socratic method went back and forth with the addition of tumor plop, pericardial knock, and an S2 split in the differential diagnosis. This would lead to further discussion of the diseases that may be associated with the aforementioned diastolic sounds and whether congestive heart failure (CHF) could be a manifestation of such illnesses? If the answer was yes, "How could you distinguish them using the history, exam, chest x-ray and an EKG?" he would continue.

All our jaws would drop, and the discussion would start and extend into multiple layers.

"Dr. NN, the ER is loud sometimes and when the patient has tachycardia, I can't tell S3 from S4 from summation gallop?"

"What about edema on the exam instead to diagnose CHF?"

He would answer calmly, "Interesting point. What is an S4? What type of edema? Was it unilateral or bilateral? How do you know how long it has been there? What are the other causes of edema besides CHF and how can you distinguish them?"

We would be mesmerized with the depth of his knowledge. The discussions would show us how little we knew, but if were willing to spend time, he would help us teach ourselves. Over time, we would use the library to find out if one part of the history or physical exam or even a lab value was better at predicting CHF than something else was. Yes, this was long before BNP (brain natriuretic peptide) became available as a blood test to potentially diagnose CHF and well before the JAMA Rationale Exam Series on congestive heart failure made us realize the importance of the history and physical exam. If the problem was identified correctly—meaning we as a group were confident that this was CHF and not pneumonia, interstitial lung disease, pulmonary emboli, or a host of other conditions—then the process would repeat itself for the next card.

Now we understood why the problem needed to remain the same, but the diagnosis could change. This was a simple yet brilliant way to provide cost-effective care for our patients without ordering every test under the sun and subsequently guessing at what to do with the results. This bastard was brilliant!

I would much later understand the concept of evidence-based medicine using pretest probability, likelihood ratios, and post-test probability, and how Dr. NN was laying the foundation for years to come. We always left morning report high on caffeine and knowledge. Armed with this knowledge, even rounding with our pretending physician (not you, Harvard) and his or her "agree with above notes" could not harm the patient. If your lead card was accepted from beginning to end, you felt as if you had just won the Nobel Prize for medicine.

Dr. NN and I would have a love/hate relationship for years to come. Although I didn't realize it at the time, he would become my mentor. Dr. NN hoped for an uncompromising set of principles guiding our training through fears and tears. Our dreams and his hopes were the same: our journey was our destination.

28

Medicine Intensive Care Unit

Elephant medicine

The second year of my residency was in full swing. I had already met the Nazi regime, the Fascist regime, and of course the Dr. NN regime. By now, we had all read *House of Gods* and realized we were living through history that was repeating itself. The Medicine Intensive Care Unit (MICU) rotation was no exception. Depending on your point of view, you either loved the MICU or hated the MICU.

Some residents loved the MICU because you didn't have to take a daily history or an admission history on an intubated patient! The residents were also happy that the patient couldn't complain, and thus the chance of having to explain yourself to the higher-ups was a big fat zero. The MICU was a favorite for adrenalin junkies and those who liked to fix numbers. You were always taking care of the sickest patients in the hospital, and your intervention for a particular ventilator setting and/or laboratory abnormality would instantly tell you whether you were a genius—or about to become a goat.

We practiced experience-based medicine in the MICU, and the evidence for our intervention wasn't always consistent. In defense of the MICU, it was difficult to make evidence-based decisions when the patient's life was at stake and time was of the essence. As such, we did more of everything than we needed to. More consults, more blood work, more imaging, and more rounding, sometimes two to three times a day.

Unfortunately, with more comes less. There was less supervision, less discussion, and less continuity. In fact, it was not uncommon in our MICU of sixteen patients for one resident to know beds one, four, and eleven thoroughly since he or she had admitted those patients, yet just know the labs and ventilator settings on the rest of the patients. Did you notice I said the bed numbers, not names? Regrettably, we often didn't have time for names.

The summary of the patients was essentially the same day after day. *CHF exacerbation in one is about the same; cardiology says we need to increase his Lasix. Urosepsis in four is not looking good, still on pressors, nothing to drain per imaging, cultures are still cooking. Eleven? Ah, who's in eleven? Oh yes, the patient with AIDS and disseminated Mycobacterium Avium Complex (MAC) and Histoplasmosis (Histo). Staying the course, Infectious Disease (ID) says we should still keep Cytomegalovirus (CMV) in our differential, although Gastroenterology (GI) doesn't want to scope him in his current condition.* MICU was the leader in abbreviations, both in conversations and on the chart.

Every day in the MICU was a model of shift work. The goal was to get the patient through another day until the next team came on board. Since patients were seriously ill, every subspecialist was seeing the patient. Let's do the math. The MICU team had three residents and three interns (one team on call every third day), four medical students (whatever), one acting intern (a bad actor, if you asked me), the MICU fellow (hit or miss, just like the one on other rotations) and the pretending (young and fresh out of fellowship.) So the MICU team, which was directly in charge of the patient, had eight MDs and five dazed and confused hopefuls. Since in theory, half the admissions were "septic," and thus diagnosed with sepsis, fill in the blanks with one of the standard answers: *This patient is headed for _____. I think this patient is _____. There is not much in the literature about____. Although trials with APC and other anti-inflammatory modalities are promising, _____ continues to be a diagnosis with more questions than answers...*

Did we have any formal training on how to break bad news to a family? No. Did a single fellow or pretending ever give us a theoretical lecture on death and dying? No. Why not? Unfortunately, it was just a continuum of the culture from the days of *House of God*. My residents, fellows, and pretendings were never taught those things, so why should I be taught things less relevant than daily labs and ventilator settings? Besides, it's better to learn by doing and figuring it out on your own, right?

Even Dr. NN was an example of this. If he had to walk uphill through snow both ways back in the 1800s, then everybody else was going to do the same. His methods weren't always pleasant, but at least his heart was in the right place, unlike my other teachers. We had forgotten what was important, and our actions lacked humility. Without realizing it, we had become robotic monsters. I didn't blame anyone, but I felt dazed and confused. I wasn't even a medical student anymore. How could this still be happening? Why were there no discussions in the MICU about the whys?

Why did we need a CT scan for a lipase elevation when we didn't think the patient was suffering from pancreatitis? We would learn years later that someone asked this question. Why did we need an echo on a patient with a murmur to rule out endocarditis without any other peripheral signs or risk factors to suggest the diagnosis? Why did we always order a renal ultrasound for an elevated creatinine that was acute and improving in a patient unlikely to have obstructive uropathy? Why did we need a daily chest x-ray on patients in the MICU? And finally, why did it seem as if no one cared?

I hope you don't misunderstand. There were times when perhaps someone cared or felt something, but those times were the exception and not the rule. And when the poster child for questioning everything—that would be me—brought something up, it was dismissed. I thought the entire process of education was to grow and learn by asking questions when you were confused. I thought the idea was to challenge your educators and hope to improve. As usual, I was wrong. The idea was unfortunately to survive and practice "monkey see-monkey do" medicine while keeping your mouth shut.

In time, I started to call my MICU rotation elephant medicine. There was a lead elephant that everyone followed without questioning. We were just going in circles with no beginning, no end, and most importantly, no purpose. Individuality was not permitted and no one would ever break free from the herd. I was just as guilty as the rest. In the beginning, I would speak up. After a while, for self-preservation, my voice became silent, and I became one of the elephants. I've already used the phrase enough, but you're thinking what I was thinking over fifteen years ago: one day…

29

Patel Humor

Will the real Patel please stand up?

When you couldn't change your work environment or the people around you, survival was often dependent on a sense of humor. Misery loves company, and what kept us going were the stories of "No way! You're lying. That really happened?" In an especially stressful rotation like the MICU, stories for me were the oxygen that allowed me to breathe, since it seemed at times I was in more need of ventilator support than my intubated patients.

One particular story of sanity-saving humor comes to mind. Think: "Will The Real Slim Shady Please Stand Up?" In this case, Slim Shady was Patel, an extremely common last name in India, especially in the state of Gujarat where I was born. Before you get excited, my last name is Mehta, not Patel. No, Patels and Mehtas are not the same. And finally, always remember all Gujaratis' Mantra (unless you're a Patel of course): "All Patels are Gujaratis, but not all Gujaratis are Patels." Since my residency training was pre-9/11, I knew plenty of foreign medical graduates, and many of them were Indian. At least by perception, a large number of these residents originated from the state of Gujarat. If the United

States will always be known as the home of the brave, then Gujarat will always be known as the home of the Patel.

As it turned out, my MICU rotation was a buffet with all the dishes named Patel. The Dazed and Confused (DC) was Patel. The intern was Patel. The fellow was Patel. Fortunately, the attending was not named Patel. It was not uncommon for members of the ancillary staff, including the respiratory tech and the nurses, to also be of Indian descent. As such, everyone who was Indian was labelled Patel. It didn't matter what part of India the "Patel" was originally from. *Really? Do we all look the same? Have you not seen my nose? I'm special! I'm a Mehta!*

So, even if you just had one doctor of Indian descent and a nurse of the same origin, the humor was already built in.

"Dr. Patel, can you please sign the order to discontinue isolation?"

"My name isn't Patel. It's Mehta."

"Oh, sorry, Doctor."

"No problem, Nurse Patel."

"But my name isn't Patel. I'm Kokila Bhanumati Subramanian, but my friends call me Koki."

Now imagine the confusion when you already had multiple doctors named Patel added to a mix in an environment where anyone who was brown was Patel! Since the MICU was busy, we were often paged, at times using the overhead speaker.

"Dr. Patel to MICU STAT!"

Like a Pavlovian dog, I showed up. "Yes, what do you want now?"

"Oh sorry, Dr. Mehta, I didn't page you, I paged the real Patel!"

I didn't know whether to laugh or cry. The one time I answer to "Patel" out of habit, they knew my real name! As I tried to make up my mind on the next course of action, DC

Patel showed up.

"I'm just a medical student and can't help you. Why are you paging me overhead?" said DC Patel.

"I didn't page you, I paged Dr. Patel, and you're not a doctor!"

This was awesome. I was already halfway to the floor when the intern Patel showed up. "You paged?"

"Not you!" screamed Koki. "I meant the real Dr. Patel!"

I couldn't resist. "But Nurse Patel, he's real."

"My name is Koki, Dr. Mehta, and this isn't the real Patel!"

"No," I said, now continuing the "Who's on first?" routine from Abbott and Costello. "You don't understand. I'm not the real Patel, but this is the real Patel."

"No, no, no!" Koki now sounded like a mad Patel. "I meant the Fellow Dr. Patel!"

The DC Patel and intern Patel turned at once like twins and walked in the other direction, disgusted. This is when the Fellow Patel walked in.

"You paged? Sorry, I was busy with the admission from the emergency room."

"Oh, so you're the real Patel?" I said. I couldn't help myself.

"What are you talking about, Mehta?"

Before I could start, Koki interrupted, "Please, doctors, be quiet! The family of patient in bed thirteen wants to talk to you about how the patient is doing. They are waiting in the family conference room."

To which the Fellow Patel replies, "I'm too busy. Send in the intern Patel!"

By now, I was beside myself and thought I would burst. I regained my composure and threw in one more jab as I turned to leave. "Is the patient in thirteen named Patel or is it

Mehta? Just want to make sure we send in the right doctor."

In moments like this, there were no hopes, fears, dreams, or tears—just laughter, and lots and lots of it. Laughter is the best medicine not only for the patient, but interestingly enough, equally necessary (and cost-effective) for doctors, too.

30

The Consult Service

Welcome to the good life.

Unlike the intern year when I did as I was told without asking any questions, I had some minor—key word being minor—perks as a second-year resident. One perk was to be assigned to the consult service. The first advantage: NO CALL!

"Surely you're not serious?"

"Yes, I am, and don't call me Shirley," was our standard line when we learned that our schedule included no call. This was for an entire month. Imagine clean underwear (don't ask), brushing your teeth (I used to think a Tic Tac was toothpaste), and of course, a shower and a shave (the Don Johnson look from *Miami Vice* would have only worked with teal scrubs, but alas, ours were green).

Yes, consult service was the good life. Work was 7 a.m. to 7 p.m. And at the end of the day, I actually went home! Every day! Say goodnight to somebody! And eat healthy! Well, let's not go crazy; I still ate nachos for dinner, a habit borne of superstition from my intern call days to avoid receiving too many admissions. The other beauty of consult service: the consults usually came from interns on other services.

I remember calling consults as an intern. It was usually a one-sided conversation with what appeared to be an issue with the telephone service because there were so many abrupt disconnections. What goes around comes around. No call and the opportunity for intern beat-downs.

It got better. On the consult service, you weren't responsible for the admission history, physical exam, or discharge summary. There were no direct patient responsibilities because you weren't part of the primary team.

I loved receiving calls from nursing meant for someone else.

"Doctor, Doctor, your patient in 3A1 bed 2 is constipated."

"I'm sorry, you want Patel, and this is Mehta. I'm not the primary team."

The consult service was busy, but it was like having a gift that kept on giving. Given the busy nature of most consult services, there were multiple residents on the service. You guessed it: divide and conquer. What the attending doesn't know (not you, Harvard) won't hurt him. So, one resident could go home early every day and one could come in late every day. If rounds were at 8:00 a.m., I could come in late and another resident would be the early bird.

The attending would ask, "Where is Mehta?"

Early Bird would reply, "We got swamped with consults. He is seeing a patient we will check out to you tomorrow."

Actually, Mehta was sleeping at home. What about the next day? You see the thing is . . . how should I put this? Let me just come out and say it: Attendings usually walk around in a myxedema coma and have a bad memory. If I was asked about the consult the next morning, I would just reply, "Oh, sorry, they changed their mind and sent the patient home." Now, we didn't do this every day, but we added enough variety to the routine to make ourselves visibly invisible. "Oh, Mehta is in clinic," Early Bird would say. Rarely would the pretending remember that clinic was only once a week, and that I'd already been in clinic twice that week.

We covered each other's backs and actually got some well-deserved R&R. Was this ethical, you might ask? I might reply: did you want me to be your doctor after thirty-six hours without sleep? Besides, all this manipulation usually gave us only a sixty-hour work week. How nice! Welcome to ClubMed.

Yes, the perks kept coming. Every consult service had a fellow who was essentially in charge of the patient's care. After all, there was no Direct Observed Therapy (DOT) for myxedema for the pretendings yet. The advantage? If the pretending took his Synthroid and started asking too many questions, the fellow would always step in. "I told Early Bird, I mean Worm, I mean Mehta, he could take care of some loose ends on other patients, sir. He's doing a great job." The fellow was actually thinking, *I'm not sure Mehta is doing a good job, but our service is very busy and we're all tired. We cover for each other and this is our fraternity honor code. We don't lie to you every minute of every day, but because liars should have good memories, we have memories like an elephant, unlike you my dear pretending.*

Yes, the consult service was like celebrating your birthday every day for an entire month. If the primary team called the consult service with a question about a diagnosis, it was easy because each consult service had the famous—I call it infamous—Six Pack. No, not the Brad Pitt Six Pack (my current buzzword for an acute rigid abdomen with peritoneal signs). I meant the six tests I could order to keep everyone busy.

In academia, the trick is to sound smarter than you really are and order a bunch of tests to do a few things. Why? 1) To keep others busy and reading in the library to figure out what was wrong with the patient; 2) We're in academia, so let's order anything and everything and think about the most ridiculous possibilities (I'm still looking for that first case of pancreatitis from a scorpion sting! Or Vitamin A intoxication from polar bear meat presenting as hypercalcemia. Though there aren't too many Eskimos in Houston. Maybe I just trained in the wrong part of town—the warmer side); 3) Billing is good; 4) If you didn't do anything, you were dumb and didn't know anything. Years later, I know better, but back then. . . .

Now that you understand the rationale, let's get back to the Six Pack. So, if I was on the nephrology consult service and the patient had nephrotic syndrome, a significant loss of protein in their urine, the Six Pack represented the six tests that I could order to keep everyone busy. It was like being at McDonald's: *Let's see. I'll take an ANA, HIV, RPR, Hepatitis Panel, Complements, and of course SPEP/UPEP, and the renal ultrasound with venous Doppler.* Oh, that's seven tests, you say? Well, you know I have a frequent customer card here. I get the seventh test for free.

I know you don't know why I'm recommending the venous Doppler, and frankly neither do I. It just makes me look smart and you stupid for not thinking about renal vein thrombosis presenting as nephrotic syndrome. Don't tell anyone this but I've been asked to order the Doppler for a while and I haven't seen it change a patient outcome without a renal biopsy, but hey, monkey see, monkey do.

If we were on cardiology, the Six Pack theme continued. Since our chairman was a cardiologist and there was so much coronary artery disease, we had to be more creative. Any monkey can order an echo, holter, MUGA, cardiac cath, and stress test, but here we had to appeal to "back in the day." We often wondered if our pretendings graduated from medical school in this century. The new generation rounded on tests that were ordered without a pretest probability. The "old school" pretendings were good with and demanded excellent physical exam skills, because frankly they didn't have that many tests they could order "back in the day". Yes, we would feed the graybeard pretending the detailed exam findings, especially related to the heart murmur. Of course, we knew the echo result about what type of heart valve deformity the patient had before the BS started.

"And Dr. Heart, what I found interesting was that there was no x descent in this patient with what I believe to be severe tricuspid regurgitation given the location of the murmur and the fact that the murmur got louder with inspiration. I was wondering, Dr. Heart, in your vast experience if you have seen pulsatile varicose veins as a manifestation of severe tricuspid regurgitation?"

We obviously had to take our Phenergan before such a presentation since the amount of nausea from this gamesmanship would otherwise have turned into vomiting. The attending's response, you ask? Well, I told you already he forgot to take his Synthroid. If he did, we let the peacock strut his feathers until he returned to the previous state of nirvana known as myxedema. Did I tell you that thyroid function tests were part of the endocrine consult service Six Pack? Oops, I must have forgotten to take my own Synthroid.

31

Coronary Care Unit LBJ

Meet Dr. Kingsley.

Alas, consult month did not last forever. It was time for what was arguably the busiest rotation during my internal medicine residency: the CCU, Coronary Care Unit. I called it the Crash Cart Unit or the Constantly Coding Unit because, well, it just seemed as if our patients were constantly trying to die. The unit was headed by a cardiology attending of Indian origin from South Africa with a thick British accent. I knew Indians traveled well, but this was ridiculous. Gandhiji was too obvious and frankly too easy of a pseudonym for this pompous, arrogant guy. So, naturally my hyperactive mind came up with Dr. Kingsley, in honor of Sir Ben Kingsley, who played Gandhiji in the Oscar winning movie of the same name. Now that I think about it, he even had a mole like Sir Ben did on his face.

The problem with Dr. Kingsley was that he was brilliant and he knew it. Although he was a researcher prior to coming to LBJ, his training was under the British system in South Africa, one that required immense clinical skills, especially in cardiology. During his training, he wasn't permitted to just order any test he desired, and thus neither could we. He was the first attending who was actually practicing evidence-based medicine (EBM) during my training who didn't realize he was practicing EBM. For him, there was a right way to practice cardiology (his way) and the wrong way (everyone else's way).

I had formed the impression that my CCU rotation would be a cakewalk, other than the hours which sucked. Think about it: How many tests are there in cardiology? Echo, holter, stress, cath: the Fantastic Four. The problem was that Dr. Kingsley needed a two-page history and physical exam to provide justification for every single test. I thought the standard indications were as follows:

1) Echo – assess left ventricular (LV) function (translation: patient is short of breath and I'm too tired to think).

2) Holter – history of arrhythmia with syncope (translation: history sucks and I'm too tired to think).

3) Stress test – chest pain (translation: cover my butt because Jim Adler, the tough smart lawyer, is never too tired to think).

4) Cath – see # 1-3 (translation: at my other training hospital, we did cath on everyone because we were too tired to think).

Everyone in the CCU had chest pain, shortness of breath, or syncope along with known risk factors for coronary artery disease including diabetes mellitus, hypertension, hyperlipidemia, and smoking. In my mind, this meant ordering at least the first three tests and considering the fourth. I was so tired of being wrong during residency, but once again I was wrong. At least I was consistent.

Here was the typical conversation with Dr. Kingsley on rounds:

Me: "Dr. Kingsley, we have a new admission with Congestive Heart Failure."

Kingsley: "You haven't killed him yet?"

Me: "Excuse me?"

Kingsley: "I assume you gave him Lasix last night?"

Me: "Yes."

Kingsley: "So, how could Lasix kill someone with CHF before I show up?"

Me: "Hypotension?" *(Sound confident, Niraj. I think Kingsley eats vegetarians like you for breakfast and may be related to Dr. NN.)*

Kingsley: "How do you collapse five liters of intravascular volume with a single dose of Lasix?"

Me: "I don't understand, sir?" *(Great, Niraj, you gave him an opening. Goodbye Mom and Dad. Next rebirth, here I come.)*

Kingsley: "You don't understand the question, English, or frankly all of the above and beyond? Damn, you don't know a bloody thing? He doesn't know a goddamn bloody thing does he?" Followed by a menacing glance at the rest of team.

You mean me? I said to myself. Silently I was hoping the suddenly deaf and mute members of the team would stop staring at the floor or ceiling, and say something to rescue my butt from certain death. I was too young for rebirth. Of course, no one came to my aid, and instead the reality continued.

Me: "I'm sorry, sir."

Kingsley: "You're sorry, but your patient should be sorry, for you could have killed him with your Lasix. Do you know how? Do you? Do you?"

Me: "No sir, but I'll find out."

Kingsley: "Good, because he survived the death test. You didn't think about it and he didn't die so Lasix wouldn't have killed this patient, but it might kill your next patient."

So, off I went to the Jesse Jones Library to learn about preload and afterload and CHF. As I continued to read, I learned about how the patient could actually have pericardial effusion (fluid in the sac that surrounds the heart) which may be misdiagnosed as CHF, especially by a novice like me. As the lump in my throat enlarged, I read that the most dangerous and severe form of pericardial effusion, known as cardiac tamponade, could actually worsen with Lasix treatment. Because these patients essentially had a tight pericardial sac, the left side of the heart was relying on preload in the form of volume from the right side of the heart. In theory, overzealous use of Lasix could diminish preload necessary for the left side of the heart.

I had my answer. I came back the next day and Dr. Kingsley, after listening to what I thought was a brilliant answer, asked me about Beck's triad and how it didn't always apply and why not. Again, I scurried back to Jesse Jones, earning imaginary frequent flyer miles, for more information about the limitations of Beck's triad. I discovered that Beck's triad was originally proposed for patients with acute trauma-induced cardiac tamponade rather than the chronic/impending cardiac tamponade more commonly seen in Internal Medicine.

Again, Dr. Kingsley was not happy. His follow-up question to the previous follow-up question was, "What is another possible scenario where the use of Lasix could kill a patient with CHF?"

Did Dr. Kingsley have a brother who ran morning report and a sister who headed the cafeteria? I once again made the journey back to my home away from home, the Jesse Jones Library. Armed with new knowledge, I returned to the CCU and told Dr. Kingsley that Lasix could be dangerous in theory in patients that had EKG changes suggestive of ongoing inferior wall ischemia. In these patients, there was a possibility that the ischemia could involve the right side of the heart, since the same blood vessel (the right coronary artery) also supplied the inferior wall of the left side of the heart in a majority of patients. If this was confirmed by a right-sided EKG showing ST segment elevation in lead V4R, it would be dangerous to use Lasix even if the patient was noted to have pulmonary edema. Once again, decreasing the preload could be harmful to these patients. The treatment of such patients, erroneously thought to need Lasix, was actually fluids with incremental adjustments based on their central venous and pulmonary pressures.

I even took it one step further. "And Dr. Kingsley, this is especially important at LBJ because we don't have a cardiac cath lab at this hospital. Time is muscle, as you have taught us."

He finally gave me the Bell's palsy half-smile.

Between the hours spent performing research at Jesse Jones and taking call in the CCU, there was little time for anything else. There were days when I didn't go home, and my car became my bed. By the end of the month, I had lost twenty pounds, making me one of the few residents who actually went down a scrubs size. In fact, I started to look like Gandhiji fasting to protest British rule. In this case, it was South African rule, but the protest was involuntary.

However, I now knew about every heart murmur imaginable, and how each murmur changed with different maneuvers. I could tell you all the wave forms of JVP, and the signs of heart disease outside the heart. Most importantly, I understood the value of self-learning, and how to think. So, Dr. Kingsley, thank you for your Emmy-worthy performance well before "House" became a household name on television. House even has an accent just like you. No mole though, sorry.

Dr. Kingsley showed me that what one knows and doesn't know is knowledge. Through all the fears and tears during my CCU rotation which I barely survived, I hoped and dreamed that someday I'd be as good as you, Dr. Kingsley, and carry forth your message of evidence-based medicine and learning by asking questions.

32

Clothing

Fat-Denial Scrubs

Since every rotation was busy—some unreasonably so like the aforementioned CCU—time was the most important commodity. It was especially important to the triple threat known as me, myself, and I. What can I say? Being selfish was a survival instinct. My goal was to maximize by minimizing. I tried to take shortcuts with every aspect of my personal hygiene. "Tic Tac" might as well have been my middle name, since brushing teeth was, well, time consuming. But then again, I could have had many other middle names, such as Speed Stick or English Leather. Don't laugh—my budget was tough.

The biggest time saver was clothing. Who had the time to shop? Clearly not a second-year resident. Knowing my luck, I was afraid that someone would collapse at the Galleria mall and my guilt gene would kick in. As a result, I would have to intervene and play doctor. Don't hate me; all residents harbored the same thoughts during their valuable time off. With no time for shopping or laundry, our attire of choice was scrubs.

To paraphrase *A Tale of Two Cities*, scrubs were the best of clothes and the worst of clothes. Let's start with the best first. If you've ever worn scrubs, you know that they're the most comfortable clothing ever made. Wearing scrubs almost makes you feel as if you're walking around naked, but covered at the same time. I would've been happy walking around in my birthday suit. After all, half of our patients had the peek-a-boo gowns with the natural air conditioning opening in the back. I don't think my department would have been too happy seeing me *au naturale* even if I told them that there was an Indian Yogi in Oregon who did exactly that.

The scrubs were not only comfortable, but they had a built in "stain blender" feature. The dark green ones seemed to take in stains particularly well. We seemed to wear our stains with pride. After a while, I was no longer sure as to the original source of the stain and began to play "Name That Stain" in my head.

A portion of my scrubs were darker from the chronically absorbed stain that had not been washed. Was that Diet Coke or coffee? Perhaps it was a bit of fluid from some cavity of the patient. Or was it nacho cheese? And there was that patient in the ER from three weeks ago who had Code Brown—stool everywhere. Nah, that couldn't be. It smelled like English Leather. Wait, a friend told me English Leather smells like shit. I was wearing shit!

It was only when it reached this point that I decided to wash my scrubs. This was the other bonus of scrubs: You could always have the hospital wash your scrubs. Free laundry service! I could do it on my own, but who had the time? Yes, I could go to my mom's house, but who needs the guilt and constant reminders from an Indian mom that someone's daughter is the same age as me. Yes, Indian moms were no different than Indian aunties when it came to constant matchmaking.

The scrubs checklist: Comfortable, check. Color absorbent, check. So far two for two. As an extension of comfort, scrubs were always a bit baggy. This allowed one to pack on a few extra pounds without anyone noticing. I'm being kind when I say a few extra pounds. It was more like a few extra pounds a month, unless you were in the CCU. Since the residency was thirty-six months, well, do the math. That's right. No one was going to call me "healthy" —I mean fat— because I had my Fat-Denial Scrubs on.

You became so dependent on scrubs that you couldn't live without them. It was not uncommon to visit the grocery store on your days off proudly wearing scrubs. Galleria mall, assuming no codes? No problem, scrubs it is. Who knows, maybe a cute Indian girl, hopefully not known to my parents and not on some matrimonial advertisement in the local Indian paper (this was before Shadi.com) would think, "Look, a doctor in scrubs!"

The problem with scrubs, however was that they made us comfortably numb. We went to restaurants in scrubs. I knew guys who went on dates in scrubs. Since we wore green all the time, at times we bought other green clothing that we would've never thought about buying otherwise. I still own— Indians are not allowed to throw away old clothing—a green sweater and a green Adidas t-shirt that came in every other color imaginable, but I wanted green. I could've bought any other color, but I chose green as if I were a freaking leprechaun. I have now given both of my prized possessions to my parents. Sadly, they still wear them as if I bought them yesterday.

Why couldn't we get dates? Because we were fat but didn't realize it in our Fat-Denial Scrubs. I once went to my mom's house with my scrubs and she thought I had a curry stain on my scrubs. *No, Mom, that's not curry, but now that I'm here, could you do my laundry and make some curry?*

I have come full circle now. I wear a coat and tie to work every day and hope my students and residents will do the same. Alas, no such luck—they wear their scrubs with a badge of honor. Some habits are hard to break, I guess. After all, I still wear my scrubs around Pearland on the weekend, hoping I won't run into a student or a resident.

33

Halfway Home

Glass is half empty or half full?

Could it really be true? It was January 1995, meaning I was halfway through my residency. The word "half" stuck in my head. Half of my patients seemed to get better in spite of me, and I still wasn't sure if the other half got better because of me. Half of my personality seemed to be a kind, gentle soul who wanted to help those less fortunate at the county hospital. The other half wanted to lock the doors to the hospital so no more patients could be seen. Half the ER was empty one day because the bus that usually came to LBJ, bus number 1, was half an hour late. Half my residency class was getting fatter but didn't know it because of the leprechaun scrubs. The other half of the class was on a weight loss program called residency training in internal medicine. Half the residents now had a steady significant other, were engaged, or had gotten married. The other half was flashing the "I'm a doctor, let's have sex" smile at every opportunity.

Depending on your point of view, the glass was half empty or half full. My associative brain then zeroed in on the idea of "full." Everyone was full of crap. The pretendings led the crap parade because, as the name suggested, they were good actors, pretending to know it all. Next in the parade came the residents, including me, because we thought we knew it all. Then came the nursing staff, because they knew what was best for the patient. The patient was full of . . . well, because some of them were constipated from all the medications that they were taking.

We were all part of a metaphorical stool asylum. The hospital was full of "bright smile" administrators who came straight out of *Leave it to Beaver*. "Golly gee, Dr. Mehta, I know you're full of crap and as you know, so am I, but let me see what I can do to alleviate some of the crap your patient is going through at this point in time." We were all singing a paraphrased Al Jarreau song:

"...And we're in this shit together, we got the kind that lasts forever"

The beds were full of patients. There were four patients to a room with many more scattered in the hallways. Sadly, everyone—except for the patient who was already occupying the bed—was selfishly hoping that someone would vacate the bed on the ward service upstairs to improve the congestion in the ER and the hallways. Doctors were full of caffeine. The cafeteria was full of Nazis. The nursing staff members were full of accents no one could understand during a code. The operating rooms were full of surgeons operating twenty-four hours a day. Their beepers were full of unanswered pages, usually from internal medicine residents like me being full of ourselves and trying to transfer patients to surgery.

The entire scene was a mixture of books I had read over the years. In front of my eyes every day was a living world straight from *1984, Ward Number 6, Lord of the Flies, Catch 22,* and of course *House of God.* At moments, we acted like dogs, so perhaps this was *House of Dogs.* And yet in between those moments, like during my fifteen minutes of solitude before rounds that I would discover years later, I felt all that was right at this place. At the time, we were just too young and too blind to see it. There were obviously daily tears from lives lost. There were also fears, stemming from multiple sources of possible repercussion that could arise as a result of the loss (remember my litigation as a third-year medical student). But the glass half full contained hopes and dreams that could never be emptied no matter how hard we tried. It was as if The County engulfed you, and while you were in it, you hated every minute of it. And yet, when you were away from it even on your rare day off, you missed it.

Over time, this had become my home. It was my house of hopes and fears, dreams and tears.

34

I Am Still Hungry

Egg drop soup, half and half, fried-only potatoes

Although half my residency was over, I still had time for more observations. Working at The County was like watching your favorite movie that happened to be a combination of comedy, tragedy, drama, romance—I lost count of how many doctors dated nurses—and horror combined into one over and over again. Every time you saw the movie, there was something new you learned, loved, hated, despised, appreciated, or became indifferent to again. Hell, if they added a song and dance with multiple wardrobe changes, it would've been a Hindi movie! But then again, none of us could sing or dance and we all wore scrubs. This explains why there haven't been too many Bollywood movies with The County theme.

Let's start with the cafeteria as an example of keen—and perhaps did-you-take-your-Prozac?— observations. When I started work, food was food. As a vegetarian, my choices were already limited, and I wasn't going to be the Indian poster child who brought tiffin packed by his mom every day. We already had Patel for that.

We had once asked a student to pick up food for the team from the local restaurant, Kim Son, in downtown Houston, about a ten-minute drive from LBJ. We later abandoned the idea when our student showed up three hours later claiming all kinds of Gulliveresque stories to account for his tardiness. So, it was the cafeteria or bust.

During my intern year, I simply ate food. There was little thought given to the meal. Down the hatch it went. Just a form of sustenance. I described it as eggs, toast, and potatoes. As time passed, my intake of caffeine increased and I believe, as a result, so did my wired observations. I had never noticed before that the eggs were runny. The toast seemed to be half toasted and half untoasted. The hash browns had a fried crisp top layer, but the rest was semi-cooked.

When I was in full caffeine mode after being awake for twenty-four hours, I grabbed bre-lun-er before morning report with you know whom. Bre-lun-er was my version of breakfast, lunch, and dinner combined into one, since it was not uncommon to have time to eat only once a day. The safest bet was the morning hours, and that usually meant breakfast.

One day, I ordered a Nazi two-for-one special. My favorite Nazi was serving breakfast, and I would later that morning be served *as* breakfast to the morning report Nazi. Although this was a bad combination, in the mind of an Indian, there's no such thing as a bad two-for-one special. I looked at my options for ordering and decided to give it a go.

Me: "Good morning, Adolph."

Breakfast Nazi: "You know my name ain't Adolph."

Me: "Right, right, you're always right, Adolph." (The last part under my breath)

Breakfast Nazi: "I can still hear you, Patel."

Calling any Indian "Patel" is basically fighting words. Sorry to all my Patel friends, but it's true. The music was already starting in my head: "Are you ready to rummmmmmbbbbbbllllllllle!" Hell, yeah. It was on.

Me: "Fine, fine. I'll just have the egg drop soup."

Breakfast Nazi: "We don't have egg drop soup for breakfast, lunch, or dinner. I've been working here for years and I ain't ever seen nor serve nobody egg drop soup."

Me: "But you do have egg drop soup. It's right there." I pointed to the loose, runny eggs.

Breakfast Nazi: "Them be scrambled eggs easy."

Me: "No, them be egg drop soup. See, that's easy."

Breakfast Nazi: "I been done with you. You want the eggs?!"

Me: "Let me think about it, but at least give me the half and half."

Breakfast Nazi: "The what? Milk is over there and we ain't got half and half. This ain't no Randall's".

Me: "I don't want milk, I want half and half. It's right there." Now I was pointing to the toast.

Breakfast Nazi: "Oh, you just lost your mind or acting the fool, and I ain't got time for neither. You want the half and half, damn it, I mean the toast?"

The madder someone else gets, the calmer I get. Something you should know about me the next time we meet. At this moment, it felt as if I was actually having those fifteen minutes of serenity that I mentioned earlier.

Me: "I'm so sorry, Adolph." I coughed to blur the words, covering my mouth. "I'll just have the fried-only potatoes."

Breakfast Nazi turned beyond black. *She almost looked like one of the demi-gods, Mom and Dad! They're everywhere! Even at The County! I should have never doubted you.*

Breakfast Nazi: "Oh, now I know you acting the fool and I know you mean the hash browns." She scooped some onto the plate.

Me: "I don't want half and half".

Breakfast Nazi: "I ain't givin' you half and half! Your stupid toast is over there!"

Me: "Yes, you are. The top layer on the hash browns is covered golden brown, full of grease, and delicious! The rest of it, just so you know, is half-cooked potato. You see now, half and half."

There was a long pause.

Me: "You don't see. Don't you watch *Seinfeld*? Remember the top of the muffin episode where the …."

The entire line behind me was collapsing with laughter and Kalimata, aka the Breakfast Nazi aka Adolph and perhaps aka

Rebecca de Mornay from *Seinfeld,* was done with me. She refused to serve me, and I exited through the entrance door, my signature move. I was half empty in that my stomach was growling and yet half full because I had made everyone laugh. Humor was like an instant jolt of caffeine during residency. Onward to the slaughter called morning report I went, for I was the main course and as always, the Morning Report Nazi was very hungry.

35

NN Becomes NNN

The death of Patel, lessons in math, and the birth of Niraj

The last time we met the Morning Report Nazi, I had labeled him Dr. NN, as in *non-negotiable*. Maybe it was my need for symmetry. Since childhood, I was brainwashed into listening to TRIPLE M FEVER of MUSIC, MAGIC, and MEENA on the damn Indian station that I was now addicted to. If there was an MMM, then there must be an NNN. Or, ah, hell, it was just my caffeine-driven neurosis. Regardless, I decided to rename Dr. NN. From this point forward, he would be NNN: Non-Negotiable Nazi. I could almost hear Shahrukh Khan saying this with his trademark stutter while tilting his head and probably wearing a yellow shirt (go rent any Hindi movie and you will understand).

On this day, I had no worries about x-rays, cards, and all other Murphy's Law happenings that seemed to follow me every fourth day to morning report. No, sir! I had learned to take care of that before I went to see the Breakfast Nazi. I was ready, and besides, I'd had an extra jolt of psychological caffeine—to paraphrase Prince's *Raspberry Beret*, I had walked out through the "in door" of the cafeteria. Bring it on, baby!

It was 6:50 a.m. and I was already seated. An early Indian? Now that is an oxymoron! I chuckled to myself silently, coffee in hand—and in mouth, and in my veins. NNN walked in at precisely 6:55 a.m. Pin-drop silence followed as was the routine when the Führer entered. There were four teams present with two residents on each, NNN, and the chief medical resident. Given his New Orleans upbringing, I called the chief Cajun. Ten of us were supposed to be present, although by the end of morning report, it was our version of Agatha Christie's *And Then There Were None,* with NNN the only one left alive.

NNN started the mental head count as he always did. *One, two, three*...I was wondering why Six was afraid of Seven, but kept my mouth shut.

Then NNN turned to Cajun. "I only count nine, and although from the looks of some of you that should count as two, there should be ten of us." Everyone simultaneously took a deep breath in to suck in the gut under their scrubs, thinking they were the guilty one.

NNN continued: "Who is missing? Damn it, who is missing? Did someone call you per the rules? They're supposed to call me, not you and you're not me so why should they call you unless they couldn't get a hold of me in which case per rules they're to call you but they know how to get a hold of me so unless I am dead there is no reason to call you!"

I was becoming short of breath just listening to that last fragment. *Why isn't NNN short of breath (SOB)? Wait, now I get it. Shut up, Niraj.*

"So again, why are there only nine of us here?"

Cajun was silent, but he was saved by the opening of the door right on queue. In the room was a big clock that screamed "Look at me!" when anyone entered the room. Patel, who entered the room, did not bother to look. The little second hand was already past "high noon," and it was now precisely 7:00:05 a.m. and counting. My inner voice started again. *No, Patel no! Go back! I know your parents think you have lots of births left due to reincarnation, but this is different. If you enter, you're coming to your own funeral.*

"What the f---!" said NNN, once again silencing my inner voice and thus saving me for another life. "Do you know what time it is?"

Patel was shaking like Govinda from the earthquake dance moves he made famous in the classic 1980's disco-themed Hindi movies. Or was Patel stuttering like Shahrukh did in portraying every single character he played in Hindi movies? Maybe it was both? "It is seeeevvvveeeeennnnn ooooo'clooccccckkk siiiiirrrrr!" replied the two-headed Indian movie star Govarukh, I mean Patel.

"Wrong as usual, Patel, or are you Mehta? Oh hell, it doesn't matter. You're both shit for brains. It's precisely 7:00 a.m. and 40 seconds and you entered at 7:00 a.m. and 05 seconds. You're late and you have wasted mine and everyone else's time by forcing me to go on this tirade." *Well, actually, you could just stop and we would be fine.* "Now it is precisely 7:01 a.m. and seventeen seconds." *You like that word precisely, don't you?* I was thinking, seeing Beavis and Butthead in my mind.

"Take your watch and make sure it is precisely *(he said it again, Beavis!)* set to the clock in this room, not to time in Mumbai. Hell, Mehta is here. Even he can set time correctly." *Really, did you have to go there?* "Now get the hell out of my morning report because we're precisely now three minutes and twenty-three seconds late!"

And like that, Patel was gone and dead, or as Justin Timberlake says, "Dead and gone." Either way, he (Patel, not Justin) was so young it would take another 84 million births before he….

Apparently, NNN had already said "Mehta" three

times, but I was still dazed and confused between trying to somehow keep Patel alive and getting my smartass inner voice to shut up.

"Damn it, Mehta! Earth to Mehta on Mars! Wake up. We are now precisely five minutes and three seconds behind schedule!"

"Sorry sir!" I responded and handed over my cards. We took turns being the lead sacrificial lamb, and I was Halal number one for today. He started with card number one:

"Patient is a fifty-six-year-old Black man with a problem of Congestive Heart Failure Exacerbation and a diagnosis of Atherosclerotic Heart Disease. And the card is signed. Good. No abbreviations. Less than or equal to five words in the description of the problem, and I know it is Mehta's signature because, well, I'd recognize that chicken scratch anywhere. Before we get going, tell me Mehta, do you have seizures?"

"Huh? I'm sorry, sir, I don't understand?"

"Do you have seizures?"

"No, sir."

"I just asked because your handwriting, especially your signature, looks like you're seizing while you're writing."

"Well, no more than usual, sir. I take my medicine now, and it's not even from India."

Everyone was snickering, including NNN. "I see. A smartass. I like that. Well, let's get going with the rest of the card, smartass."

What! I just got a compliment from NNN! Winner. I just hit the jackpot.

Ah, but all good things must come to an end, and my moment of euphoria lasted about fifteen seconds before my card was torn to pieces and then thrown at me with amazing accuracy. NNN was old, but he could still aim. The crumbled pieces lay on the floor like my broken spirit.

The next batter—I mean card—came up. In my mind, this card seemed to represent a simple case, but Cajun was in the habit of brown-nosing. *I have the brown nose to trump all brown noses, dumbass,* I was thinking, hoping again my inner voice would soon run out of batteries, or at least find a mute button.

Cajun always wanted to impress everyone with his knowledge of cardiology. He planned to apply for a cardiology fellowship, which at that time was considered the "God Fellowship." It should be called the Jerk Fellowship, because most guys going into that particular field were, well…and no, just in case you were thinking, I wasn't going into cardiology, but I did consider it.

Cajun decided to take my simple case and jazz it up. I paraphrased the following dialogue below as I remember it best, using a math analogy.

Cajun: "You know, NNN, I was thinking that perhaps one plus one doesn't always equal two."

NNN: "In what country?"

Cajun: "No, seriously, I'm just saying sometimes two plus two doesn't equal four."

NNN: "On what planet?"

We never liked Cajun, so when we realized that NNN was handing Cajun a shovel to dig his own grave, who were we to interfere? Breakfast and a show, remember?

Cajun: "Well, sometimes you have to use the distributive property to take into account and think about addition before subtraction. Remember My Dear Aunt Sally?"

NNN: "Hum." We got ready for another jolt of humor caffeine. "That's very interesting."

NNN: "You see, Cajun. You bring up an interesting point. The other day I was pissing in the bathroom and it thundered outside." He made a loud sound of thunder that probably awoke the sleep apnea patient in the emergency room nearby.

NNN: "Does that mean that I need to immediately call the *New England Journal of Medicine* and report a new association between thunder and my micturition stream?"

I thought the residents were going to collapse from laughter leading to an involuntary micturition incident. How would we explain to others that our scrubs appeared a shade darker for the rest of the day? But somehow we kept it together.

Cajun: "No sir, I'm just saying—"

NNN: "You know Cajun, that's your problem. You're always just saying. As to the My-Dear-Aunt-Sally bullshit, let me tell you something. Anything is possible. If I had an aunt named Sally, and I don't, but if I did and she had testicles, she would be my uncle! You see anything is possible in medicine, but what you're trying to figure out using the brain that God has given you is whether something is likely. You betting on unlikely-but-possible costs everyone, including all the taxpayers in this room, a whole lotta money and for no good reason. So, think before you order tests, and use your reasoning power. You have a brain, at least one that I know about, unless you've had a lobotomy the residency program didn't tell me about because I've told the program director I don't want shit for brains. But maybe they thought I meant no brains. Ah hell, I'm tired. Patel pissed me off and now you. Niraj did a good job today, otherwise I would have had a heart attack."

He knows my first name! Jesus Christ—I mean Holy Krishna Mom and Dad, I swear. I mean Bhagvan ka sam. I was overwhelmed with joy while Cajun was crawling out the door with one plus one testicle equals two testicles in his hand. Oh, what a wonderful world, Louie Armstrong.

Through fears and tears, I for a moment had fulfilled my hopes and dreams. I was on cloud nine the rest of the day, and as I turned the keys to start my car at 9:05 p.m. precisely, finally going home, I was smiling when it started to thunder. No, Cajun was not next to me. I burst out laughing and suddenly had an urge to pee.

36

Nursing Staff

My enemy was my only friend.

The second year of residency was almost over and I was clearly starting to understand the phrase "Keep your friends close and your enemies closer." At the time, it seemed that if you weren't a fellow internal medicine resident—excluding the MICU jerk who seemed to be everywhere at once to torment me—you were my enemy. Ah, so many people to keep close and such little time. Everything and everyone became gentle background noise when compared to every resident's mutually sworn enemy from day one, especially at The County.

The enemy, of course, was nursing. Koki was the only exception to the rule, and exceptions didn't last long at The County. She was gone well before I finished my residency. Why did we hate nurses? After all, I told you earlier that doctors and nurses were sometimes sleeping together. Sadly, sleeping together didn't mean you actually liked each other. It was simply a turf war, like surgeons and internists, except at a higher, more intense level. Nurses at LBJ had been there for years, some for decades, having transferred from the old Jefferson Davis Hospital. This was their house, and like the

Under Armour commercial, their motto was, "We must protect this house." Nurses saw doctors as trespassers who simply came to LBJ because they had to be there, and would leave as soon as they could. They were probably right, because back then and even now, how many residents who trained at a county hospital actually stayed there to become faculty?

Yes, this was nursing territory, and we weren't invited guests. From the beginning, they tested us. I'm still convinced nurses had weekly meetings during which game plans were developed to show residents who was in charge. For starters, they would constantly page you with BS. "Doctor, doctor, your patient in 3A room 4 bed 3 wants a different diet. He forgot his dentures and he wants to change to a puree diet from a soft mechanical diet, but remember he is a diabetic but with his kidney problems, doctor, as you are probably aware, doctor, from his diabetes means we can't just give him a puree with too much protein because you know too much protein is not good for him and I saw him peeing today and there is a lot of foam in his urine and I think that means he has too much protein in his urine so may be a nutrition shake but be careful because of his hypertension because we don't want to give him too much salt, but I'm sure you already knew that.

"So, just tell me what to do, because you know I'm just a nurse and you know more than me because well you're a doctor, thank you, thank you so much and sorry if I bothered you thank you again so much so you are coming now to write the order right, I mean I'm sure you know we're not supposed to take verbal orders thank you."

"First of all, stop patronizing me. Second of all, how did you say all that in a single breath? Third of all—"

My beeper went off, and it was one of her nursing buddies.

"Forget it. I'm on my way."

Once you had mastered all possible medication and diet combinations in an effort to prevent these annoying pages, nurses would just take the game to the next level. "Doctor, Doctor your patient in 3C room 8 bed 2, well his family is here and they would like to know what's wrong with him and I'm just a nurse but you are a doctor so I told them that you are a wonderful doctor and as busy as you are that you are doing a wonderful job with their loved one and that you would be coming to talk to them right?"

As if I had any choice. If I didn't go, the calls would keep coming. If I didn't go in time, next time they would page me on my call day for even worse BS. Did I mention "family" at LBJ meant an average of ten people with fifteen opinions? At the time, I was convinced at least half of them were bipolar.

Nurses drove me crazy during training, and as the phrase suggested, I tried to keep my "enemies" closer. As was the case during my Family Practice rotation in medical school, I failed to realize that nurses were the most important part of my journey. I didn't understand that nurses were often right and I was wrong. They were actually my best friends and perhaps my only friends at LBJ who didn't have hidden motives or needs. The so-called constant harassment was a simple test to see if I was one of them. I guess they had seen too many doctors hurt patients with their arrogance and attitudes of "I know best, I'm the doctor, you're just a nurse."

Hippocrates would have been proud of the nursing staff for following what I had forgotten in two short years: "Do no harm." I was slowly learning that harm came in many forms and didn't always require verbal clues. It was a starting point for me, and I would need many more years of lessons from the nursing staff to remind me that I was sometimes the enemy—to myself, to my patients, to my colleagues, and to all those around me both in and out of the hospital. If they dreamed that they could change doctors, why could I not hope to change at least myself?

$

37

I Hate Clinics

Good intention, bad consequence

My entire residency was not in the hospital. It just seemed that way. Perhaps it was because I liked being in the middle of the action and had gotten used to all the Nazis at LBJ. Perhaps patients were too healthy in the clinic. We were bored in clinic, and no one wanted to be there. However, I was required to be there one half day per week unless I was on overnight call. Since there were more months with on call responsibilities than those without, there were times when I was excused from clinic for long periods of time. How was I providing any continuity to my patients with chronic, usually progressive diseases by missing four months in a row of clinic?

Most residents hated their clinics, and I was certainly no exception. By the second year, multiple plans had been devised by different sets of residents to avoid clinic. Some plans were bolder than others. Since I wasn't a descendent of William Wallace, I didn't want to take chances clearly out of proportion to my ability to follow through on them. My plan was simple: We would pair up and show up to clinic every other week. One week, I would see all of my patients as well as those of my tag-team colleague. My friend would return the favor the following week.

If you were in clinic, you weren't on call. This meant an extra half-day off every other week. If you were in clinic, you were usually on a consult month, but as you may remember we already had the Early Bird and Owl combination for that. Patients were getting seen. The numbers looked good which made the administration happy. The things we did to have a reasonable sixty- or seventy-hour work week! As I suggested, my plan was simple, and if anyone asked about the missing resident? "Dr. Missing is in the hospital running late from a new consult, but don't worry, I will see their patient," I would reply.

What about the bolder plans? I was too chicken, but the other residents apparently liked Russian roulette. With one such plan, the resident would simply not show up on the day of his assigned clinic. He would just tell the clinic staff that he was too busy taking care of unstable patients in the hospital.

Believe it or not, there was even a higher level of boldness. Some residents would double book a patient. How could the patient show up for appointments with the continuity and pulmonology clinic if they were scheduled for the same time?

But to succeed, you had to understand the term "rarely." Just like anything else, I'm sure if anyone had the time to investigate, they would have figured it out, and the dangerous game would have been over. But who had the time? We were in the era of paper charts and simple computer algorithms. And with clinics as busy as they were with constant shifting of residents and pretendings, no one checked! It wasn't that we didn't care—or unfortunately, maybe it was. We were just so tired of being overworked, underpaid, and underappreciated. In the end, who suffered? The patients did, because as I would learn years later, all good medical care starts in clinics to prevent ER visits and by extension, admissions to the hospital. Primary care clinics are the foundation without which the rest of the system collapses.

Who else suffered? I did because I wasted an opportunity to learn, and more importantly, I failed to understand the consequences of my actions. We were exhausted, and perhaps we just wanted to have a conversation with someone, about how unfair our training was.

Instead we chose to bend the rules without realizing that we were just digging a deeper hole. Perhaps I was bitter, like the caffeine flowing through my veins, but I would need over a decade to understand that "don't ask, don't tell" was not the answer.

So many hopes and fears, dreams and tears, and yet such little time. And just like that, before I knew it, the second year of residency was over.

38

The Call Room

One-star property at best

Had two years of residency really passed by that quickly? Was I already ten years out of high school? At least now, I have the luxury of asking myself such questions. During residency, the only question that mattered was "How can I get home earlier?" Even after all the patients I had seen since my medical school days, I was confident, and yet confused. We were supposed to appreciate the beauty of gray like our attendings, but we just wanted the world to be black or white. You are either too healthy or too sick to be on my team, remember?

So two years had gone by in a flash and I could barely remember information from any of my medical school classes, certainly not the Krebs Cycle, a personal tragedy since my undergrad major was biochemistry. When are they going to get rid of biochemistry in medical school, anyway? My gift was observations, and as an extension, learning from these observations using humor and perhaps exaggerating their relevance in my own mind as a means of survival. After all, how much caffeine could one resident possibly consume in a day?

I was starting the third year of residency and had more free time, I noticed for the first time the overnight call room. I think it was only because I'd rarely frequented the call room up until that point. In time, however, I had become more efficient with patients. Instead of thirty minutes, I could admit a new patient in twenty minutes, which gave me ten precious minutes of call room time. Now I could once again afford the transient rest and relaxation that the call room supposedly provided.

I've never been to prison, but in the days of my residency, the call room was probably similar, with the exception of bars and an open toilet. The call room was small but it had just enough room for two bunk beds and a bathroom. A small, single, nondescript table sat at one end, and an equally dull but clearly screaming "empty me!" trash can sat at the other end. The mattresses resembled some of my terminally ill cachectic cancer patients, with lumps and bumps that matched the asymmetric painful lymph nodes on those unfortunate souls. The cover was a small white bed sheet. The sheet's length never did allow it to be tucked comfortably under the mattress. If I turned from one side to the other, the sheet came off. At least this took away the need for a blanket, which was usually available only on a first-come, first-served basis. Sounds like economy class to me. When was the last time anyone said, "I can't wait to fly economy class—it's so comfortable!"

What about a pillow, you may ask? What, you want a pillow or a blanket? Confused? I was too at first, but I was a third-year resident by now and had finally figured it out. You see, the blanket was the pillow. By strategically folding it, the blanket would serve as a pillow. Lucky for us, Houston was hot, and besides, we already had a blanket. I mean a sheet that covered the cadaver. I mean the mattress!

Who got the top bunk? That was easy. It was the rule

of scrubs, not first-come, first-served. If your scrub size was the same since you started residency, you got the top bunk. If it changed to XXL, you got the bottom bunk, for the safety of all involved. I actually dreamed of a fat resident crashing through the top bunk and crushing the poor intern below, but then realized this was a false dream, because interns and residents rarely shared the same call room. Besides, which intern in 1993 actually saw the call room? Well, other than that bizarre call with the peacock attending during my intern year.

In the end, these so-called rules for bed assignment were always trumped by seniority. I was now a senior resident, and I would finally have the authority to pick the top or bottom bunk. My scrubs size had remained the same thanks to the once-a-day meal known as cafeteria food, so I took the bottom bunk. I must also admit that seeing the junior resident struggle to climb up and down the top bunk multiple times a night was a source of cheap enjoyment. There was no ladder—you just got on the bottom bunk and propelled yourself to the top. I know I took some chances and for fun put the XXL junior resident on the top bunk. Maybe that's why I had that recurring dream. Back then, all I could come up with was, "What goes up must come down" and "Gravity's a bitch, isn't it?" Now I would hum John Mayer like it was my own song!

"Oh gravity, stay the hell away from me
And gravity has taken better men than me (now how can that be?!)"

The call room floor was made up of tiles as cold as my heart on call days. The lighting was minimal and matched my dark mood. Walls and ceilings were equally drab with a coat of white paint that was long overdue for cleaning, even more so than my dirty scrubs. The drawers were full of pink history and physical exam papers as well as white papers for daily progress notes. The trash can portended the future, offering an inkling of which resident may need a "stress test" to assess the possibility of coronary artery disease in the future. It contained wrappers of every type of chip imaginable: Funyuns, Cheetos, Doritos, Ruffles, Sour Cream and Onion Lay's all gave the room—and probably our breath—a unique aroma. Savory needs sweet, right? No worries: the army of chip wrappers was surrounded by wrappers from the other major food group during residency: Twinkies, mini-doughnuts, Snickers, M&M's, and Reese's Peanut Butter Cups. To this day, I'm surprised we didn't have worms making a home in our mouths. Thank God bacteria are invisible to the naked eye.

What about the bathroom? It held a small sink with stains from multiple toothpastes. Of course, I couldn't lay a claim to any of those stains. I was a Tic Tac man throughout residency, favoring green ones, of course, to match my green scrubs. At times, the mirror just above the sink seemed to be a trick mirror from Astroworld, a local Houston amusement park I had visited multiple times during my childhood. Everyone had the same confused look when it seemed as if the reflection was obviously lying. Or was it? *How did I get so thin? How did I get so fat? Are there more planets or zits on my face? Should I shave soon? I didn't know my hair could do this without hairspray.*

In the end though, the vacant, expressionless look into our own reflection suggested the same universal question that was left unanswered: "How the hell did I get here and where exactly am I going?" I have never been a fan of Adam Sandler movies or of his vulgar humor which is so often directed to toilets. As such, I will leave toilets out of this discussion. I will simply tell you that I still have nightmares about the toilets in the call room and will leave the rest of the details to your imagination.

Honestly, having a better call room was never part of my altruistic hopes and dreams for the future generation. And even if I did, today's call rooms have far surpassed my wildest dreams. There are multiple computers, flat-panel TVs, a small sofa, a shower, and a small desk. All that is missing is mood lighting—the residents have a mini-refrigerator and a microwave, and they bring their own iHome to listen to music while they type away at frantic speeds as if trying to meet deadlines.

Although I'm not grumpy and old, out of spite I admit I dream of having some of my residents—the lazy ones—spend just one night in the call room of my residency days long gone by, preferably on the top bunk. How will they ever appreciate five-star accommodations if they've never been to one-star ones? Never mind, I'm starting to sound like an Indian. Wait a minute, I'm. . . .

39

Paper Trails

Pink or white: what's your color?

The pink and white sheets of paper that seemed to be everywhere and yet nowhere when you needed them most were an integral part of my existence. We didn't have an electronic medical record system. Therefore, everything was handwritten. All admission notes were written on pink sheets of paper and served as the admission history and physical exam (H&P). All other daily notes known as the progress notes ("agree with above" notes) were written on white sheets of paper. These papers were similar in every aspect except for color. They were also lined with a small box on the bottom left corner for the patient stamp and identification information.

The papers, however, were usually found any place except where they were supposed to be. Each patient unit of the hospital had a small work area where all forms were stored. The contraption which housed these forms resembled a rectangular shoe box. Each little cubby area was labeled with a half-peeled-off sticker. Unfortunately, this was chaos theory at best. Usually the papers were not in the correct sections of the shoe box. Consent forms were placed with work excuse forms in the same area where admission H&P or progress note papers were located. Where were the pink and white sheets? Well, some were in the call room. Others had gone AWOL as if they had somehow grown legs and ran out of the hospital, a mad dash home before our chicken scratch handwriting could make its mark. *I don't remember dismissing you! Get back in here now!*

When I did find the paper, it still failed to serve its purpose. Why? For rules that I never did fully understand, you weren't allowed to write an admission H&P on the white progress note paper. You also weren't permitted to use pink paper for the daily progress note. How then could I admit sixteen patients with only twelve pieces of pink paper available and one thousand pieces of white paper? Was this BS the inspiration for the Alanis Morissette song I heard not so ironically at least five times a day from my trips back and forth from LBJ to home? Was I supposed to dye the white paper pink? Where would I find the dye? Was I supposed to cut the paper in half? If I did, was it still a legal medical record since I'd altered it? Did I mention we were already killing trees? It seemed as if everyone was writing a note, and for reasons that made no sense, the paper was not two-sided.

Have you ever seen a medical student write a history and physical exam note? It is usually eight pages long. Who can spare eight sheets of single-sided pink paper? Every day, these thoughts reverberated in my head until I came up with a solution: Hoarding. Yes, long before the A&E TV series, hoarding was the answer. Whenever I encountered extra pink sheets of paper, I placed them in my coat. Although my inner voice said "you're brilliant," all the other future Nobel Prize winners—all other residents-in-training at the time—had the same inner voice repeating the same mantra: *Hoard, Patel. If you don't, Mehta will. Hoard Patel! Hoard. It is your privilege*. So, everyone acted like a cheap, stingy, hoarding

Gujarati. For Patel and I, this came naturally because we were actually Gujaratis, the predominant group of residents originating from the Western State of Gujarat in India. Everyone else adapted and became an honorary Gujarati in my eyes.

It didn't solve the problem. How long do you think folded paper can stay in a white coat without starting to look like a piece of origami that no one could identify? You get the picture. At least it didn't fly out of our pockets like a pink swan.

You're probably wondering, "Why not just ask for more pink paper?" If so, you're brilliant. Stay away from my Nobel Prize! We did ask many times, but remember the "bright smile" administrator? The one with the tonic-clonic head moving back and forth with the notepad out every time we asked for help? *(Wait a minute—that pad isn't pink, is it?)*. He just smiled and kept his internal Al Jarreau going without supplying us with more pink paper. In desperation, we even started to trade pink paper for chips, candy bars, and even meal tickets. That approach didn't last long but added to the vending machine revenue. Now you know why vending machines used to empty so quickly at LBJ in the 1990s.

With all that I had faced in residency and the many straws that had repeatedly broken this camel's back, I now had to deal with this? This was beyond absurd. Together with my colleagues, including Patel, I decided to write on the lower portion of the page without lines. ("That is not a legal area to write, young man.") When that failed, we started to write on the back of the paper. ("That is not a legal area to write, young man.") When both sides of the paper were full, we wrote in smaller handwriting—micrographia—as if we all had early Alzheimer's. Still need more paper to write our notes? No problem, our notes just got shorter.

Although I harbored thoughts of actually cutting the

paper, I wanted no part of being the lead resident who set this precedent. *(Oh, you have the Mehta paper? That is not legal, young man, you should know that. Mehta is currently in prison and never finished his residency.)* So, what about those admissions and twelve sheets of pink admission H&P paper? What could we do when we were left paperless with more notes left to write? I actually thought about combining the usual two Lopezes or two Garcias, but that would still leave me two sheets short. Don't worry, I never actually combined them. I'm not an idiot.

Of course, we eventually decided to just write the remaining admissions on white sheets of paper. Rebel Billy Idol—that's me. Unfortunately, this was a vicious cycle, and the pendulum over time would lead to a shortage of white progress note paper. Why? If I was going to admit sixteen patients, I might as well use white sheets on all sixteen patients. Why write half of the patients' admission H&P on pink paper and the other half on white paper? And if I was going to write it on white, I made sure to stay uniform in breaking the rule—and have the intern and the medical student write on the white paper too.

We continued this practice, even when pretendings screamed at us for writing admission H&Ps on white paper. As the weeks passed, we now suddenly had a surplus of pink paper! The chart, which was already looking like Tolstoy's *War and Peace* with the addition of separate H&Ps from every member of the admit team, now had clear sections of white with shades of pink and vice versa, depending on the time of the month. Maybe we should've asked the patient to write their own H&P so we could actually figure out what was wrong with them.

Some of my dreams for the future were big. Others, not so much. I had a small dream that maybe someday I could change the color of the paper at The County to a single shade.

Alas, the dream never came true directly, but it was fulfilled indirectly. Little did I know then that the pink and white sheets of paper would, after spending so much time together, fall in love and give birth to a beautiful baby known as EPIC, the current electronic medical record system used by The County.

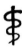

40

The Chart

The fine line between War and Peace and VSSLGFD

The medical chart was the center of everything I did for three years. All my thoughts were recorded there for eternity. The problem: as the chart became thicker, the scrutiny of its contents diminished. Who actually has the time to read *War and Peace* from cover to cover? And yet, how would I learn if no one would pay attention to my mistakes, even if the patient somehow managed to survive them? Everyone was guilty of this, but in the beginning it was easier to laugh at others and pretend all was OK with the man in the mirror. We would make fun of surgery notes and even gave these notes their own abbreviations. Surgical Attending Note: VSSLGFD (Vital Signs Stable. Looks Good From Door). Or the version that didn't need abbreviations, given its terseness: "Agree with above." Unfortunately, medicine attendings were equally guilty of the "agree with above" notes. I didn't blame them. How could cardiology attendings be asked to run the General Medicine Ward Service when the last time they led such a service with confidence was during residency over twenty-five years ago? That is, if you were lucky enough to have a clinical attending. At least clinical attendings could teach you about their particular area of expertise, and ask for consultative opinions for assistance from other specialists when the patient had problems outside the field of cardiology.

Unfortunately, not all attendings were "clinical" in training. Some attendings worked in labs and wrote grant papers for their survival in the "publish or perish" model of academia. But grants didn't always come through. Solution? Let's see. Why don't you go see some patients? It doesn't matter if you haven't practiced clinical medicine in over ten years and haven't kept up with any aspect of leading a clinical hospital team. The resident is there. You'll be fine.

Really? Fine? Would you want me to come to your lab and start running PCRs and gel amplification protocols without any experience or training? Sadly, these pretendings would stroke my ego and tell me I was the best resident they had ever worked with. I would drink up this false praise like a bottle of Petrus not realizing that it was Riunite on ice, *how nice*! I would receive great evaluations from such pretendings, and like many others before me, started to believe my own press clippings. It was only with my third year upon me that I came to realize how little I really knew, and that I was part of the grand scheme, conscious or subconscious, known as grade inflation.

My eyes were finally open and I didn't like what I saw. Your care as a patient was only as good as the lead resident or fellow taking care of you at the county hospital. There were exceptions (Harvard, NNN), but the exceptions did not invalidate the rule. I would learn years later that experience is what allows us to make the same mistake over and over again with a higher level of confidence. Sadly, I was the poster child for that statement and have hurt people over the years. I dreamed and hoped that I would be honest with my students and residents and refuse to become their "Agree with above" pretending.

41

Wake-Up Call

Stop burying your mistakes.

I was treated as a junior attending by the time I was a third-year resident. Although I was leading the inpatient team with very little supervision, what I didn't realize then was that I was only pretending to take care of my patients. NNN, however, always seemed to shock me back to reality. It was as if he was my scheduled Electroconvulsive Therapy, whether or not I thought I needed it.

When I was starting to strut like a junior peacock, NNN asked me, "Niraj, do you know why you never learn from your mistakes?"

I was thinking to myself, *because I never make any*, but I kept my mouth shut just in case the double rectum analogy was coming again. Knowing by now that short answers were best when dealing with NNN, I simply replied "No, sir."

"You never learn from your mistakes because you bury them!"

"Excuse me?" I was angry and confused, but short answers were better, remember?

"You see patients in the hospital and then you send

them out. Do you ever see them during follow-up?"

"Occasionally," I replied.

"Then how do you know what you may have done was wrong? Your patient may have gone to another hospital and died, or hell, even died at home. You see, you are burying your mistakes because you will never learn if you assume that your patients did well just because you never saw them again."

I was angry and visibly upset but answered, "Yes, sir." I couldn't move.

NNN, as was his way, replied, "What are you, a statue? Get out of here. That's all I have to say to you for now."

Like a dog with his tail between his legs, I turned around and whimpered away. Although I was upset, Kübler Ross suddenly came to mind. Perhaps I was in denial and NNN was right. What was it again? Denial, anger, bargaining, depression, acceptance. This could not continue. I was already starting to hate others, but perhaps as Mahatma Gandhiji suggested, it was time to be the change I wished to see in the world. I would have to learn the Michael Jackson way by starting with the man in the mirror. I decided that I would try to follow every patient I saw in the hospital later in my clinic. I hoped and dreamed somehow it would change me.

42

I Love Clinics

Healing Mrs. Jones, not just her disease

The change was instantaneous and much less painful than the verbal version of ECT (Electroconvulsive Therapy) that I needed but hated receiving from NNN. My patients were excited to see a familiar face in the clinic, the same one that they had seen less than two weeks ago in the hospital when they were acutely ill. They would hug me and I would melt in their arms like Silly Putty. I was their doctor, but without realizing it, they had become my psychiatrists. If they were not doing well, I could readmit them to the hospital under my service and learn from my mistakes before I buried them. If they didn't follow-up, instead of being happy *(DNS! One fewer patient to see!),* I would pick up the phone and find out why they missed the appointment. My fear was that perhaps I did bury my mistake, and that's why they didn't show up for their scheduled clinic appointment.

If I was leaving the rotation but the patient needed to be admitted to the hospital, I would admit them to the next team, but stop by to make sure the patient was OK. For the first time, I was enjoying my clinic, and I realized that all good care started in clinics. I began to understand the disconnect between the inpatient world and the clinics. The only ones suffering from confusion and lack of effective communication between doctors were the patients, whom I considered to be innocent victims of the system. Charts were getting thicker. Patients were under the care of more and more consultants. As a result, I tried hard to schedule multiple clinic visits to LBJ on the same day. A significant number of my patients had transportation issues, and required multiple buses to reach LBJ. My patient could see me in the morning for continuity clinic and then see cardiology in the afternoon. Simple and common sense. Again NNN came to mind, for he often said that common sense is not so common.

I also came to the harsh conclusion that I wasn't curing anyone of disease. I had chosen the field of Eternal Medicine. I was simply changing the slopes of eventual poor outcomes with chronic illnesses that, like a rollercoaster, would have their peaks and valleys. My heart was like a ticking clock, and as Coldplay would suggest much later, I started to wonder, *"Am I part of the cure or am I the disease?"* In reality, I was hurting patients with my arrogance and indifference. Knowledge of congestive heart failure was not enough. I needed to understand Mrs. Jones, who happened to have congestive heart failure.

It had taken me nearly seven years, starting with baby steps as a medical student, to open my eyes. What I didn't understand then was that I was finally healing human suffering. All I had to do was look into my patients' eyes and listen to their words to reflect on their hopes and fears, dreams and tears, which were not so different from my own.

43

Continuity Patient

Krishna, you changed me forever.

I still loved the adrenalin kick of being in the hospital, but it meant little without clinic follow-up and continuity. I cancelled my agreement of showing up to clinic incognito every other week, and chuckled when nurses started to wonder out loud why they saw me so often. I would give them my best Bell's palsy smile and reply, "Nah, I've always been here. It just seems that way with all the rotations I'm on." I was hoping my nose would not give away my Pinnochioesque answer.

Although I was now a seasoned third-year resident with the end of my endless training in sight, suddenly my BFF known as "clinic" reminded me that the best was yet to come. I had followed a patient I called Krishna for almost three years in clinic. Why did I call her Krishna? She had severe chronic obstructive lung disease, blue lips, a ruddy complexion, and clubbing—the changing of the angle between the nail bed and nail fold. She looked like what I had been worshiping my entire life as a Hindu. *(Yes, I know Krishna is a man, Mom and Dad. But please, this is my story.)* She was, however, far from Krishna in personality. Frankly, she should have been married to NNN. She was a crusty old crone! She had driven me crazy for three years with her refusals to stop smoking. I had tried it all. Begging, screaming, nicotine gums, pills. Hell, I had even taken the cigarette package straight out of her purse on multiple occasions and thrown it in the trash can. One time when I left, she actually retrieved it from the trash! She was on a budget, she explained.

"Stop smoking your damn cigarettes then, Krishna," I would say. "Don't you know how expensive they are?"

I had shown her pictures of "before cigarette lung" and "after cigarette lung," even drawing out diagrams of how lung function declines much faster in smokers. No success. I had shown her "smoking is glamorous" pictures of the old, withered guy I had seen in magazines and on television. I told her that would be her. Krishna politely, in her deep Lou Rawls voice, told me, "That's not me. I'm a woman."

"Damn it, Krishna, you're going to kill me," I replied once.

"Maybe you should enjoy your last days and smoke a cigarette. Want one?"

"Why do you keep coming back to torment me?" I asked her.

She replied, "Because you care and you just don't know it."

I was speechless, and if you know me, you know how rare that is.

"I what?"

"You heard me," she continued. "I've seen a lot of doctors in my lifetime, but you're the only one who hasn't given up on me. I know my lungs suck and I have that COPD or emphysema or scars in my lung or whatever and I'm blue and all these doctors comment on my funky fingers, but no one cares about me. They just care about my disease."

Who are you? I was thinking. A Shahrukh Khan Krishna who always makes people cry just like the character he portrays in Hindi movies? I gave her a spontaneous hug, tears flowing in my eyes.

One week later she came back to the clinic without an appointment. "Your favorite patient is here to see you," said one of my nurses. "Don't worry. She isn't sick, but she has a present for you."

I walked in and Krishna handed me a pack of cigarettes. "I'm not going to take up smoking, Krishna."

"It's not for you to start. I've decided to stop smoking."

A small leak started once again in the twin lakes on my face and soon there was an embarrassing puddle by my feet. This time, she initiated the hug and told me, "You're a good doctor, rough on the edges, but don't stop fighting for your patients. We are human beings, not diseases."

After what seemed like a moment that would last forever, I let go. She told me that this would be her last visit. She felt that her end was near and wanted to spend her remaining time taking care of her grandchildren. I protested, but as usual Krishna won. She wanted to exit the world on her own terms. Sadly, she died at home several months later, but she somehow lives on as a dream of why I do what I do, forever in my heart.

44

The Elderly Couple

De Nile is not just a river in Egypt.

Clinics were a constant reminder of what happens when you assume you know your patients. As an Eternal Medicine doctor, my patients were getting older, and thus I focused on diagnosing and treating depression and osteoporosis. I was in denial—consciously or subconsciously—that old people do have sex. Perhaps it's because all of us are uncomfortable with the thought of our parents doing the deed, especially for those of us of Indian origin. Indian movies from my childhood were risky if they showed a bare ankle! It also does not help if you have a gift, as I do—or is it a curse?—of instant visual imagery, even if it involves ankles. To this day I believe I was a product of Immaculate Conception.

As it turns out, I was wrong as usual about my elderly patients practicing abstinence. The patient's name was Rose because she reminded me of one of the characters from the TV show *Golden Girls*. I had been taking care of her for three years, and yes, she did have osteoporosis.

Rose came in for a routine visit and told me that she was having a discharge. Of course, with all the time I spent taking care of hospitalized patients, I was thinking postmenopausal bleeding and the possibility of uterine cancer. As usual, I was wrong. I was too shy to ask detailed questions— c'mon, man, she was like my grandmother—but started the usual work up. I was shocked to discover that Rose had a sexually transmitted disease. *"De Nile" is not just a river in Egypt,* said the inner voice. *Shut up,* I replied.

After my initial heart rate variability stabilized, I was relieved to learn that her disease was easily treatable with no long-term consequences. I broke the news to her and she responded with, "Good, I'm glad to hear that, but you better check out Jolly, 'cause he's the only one I'm doing on and off." Jolly was another patient I'd also taken care of for the past three years. He got his nickname because he was always smiling.

I was again speechless. Maybe there was an association with me being in clinic and becoming speechless, because this was the second time it had happened. I was thinking I should send this possibility to the *New England Journal of Medicine,* but Cajun wasn't around, and given the *N* of two resulting in a limited power of study, I quickly abandoned the idea.

Rose continued, "You OK, Dr. Mehta? Don't be shocked or embarrassed. Old people have sex too. Besides, this should be easy for you. Jolly is one of your patients too. In fact, I met him here in clinic waiting to see you almost three years ago!"

I was a brown Marcel Marceau for the rest of the encounter. I treated Rose and subsequently Jolly, and the couple did fine. In fact, they got married six months later at ages seventy-nine and seventy-five, and even brought wedding pictures to the clinic. I had become a matchmaker. *Ha, I say to all you Indian uncles and aunties. I'm a matchmaker without trying.*

I dreamed that maybe someday if you were in my clinic, you too could get married. Why didn't I invent an app for "dating while waiting" at the doctor's office? Oh, I forgot that such an act would not have been covered by Medicare.

45

Fellowship?

And then there was one…

I had learned so much over the last three years, yet I still felt confused. My cup of knowledge was not even half full, but residency training was almost over. What if I killed patients in the real world? There would be no ER or pretending to blame. Would Texas Hammer Jim Adler know me by name? Would I become the poster child of incompetency for the Indian community? Would all Indian uncles hate me and banish any thoughts of having me join their busy subspecialty practices?

The culture, especially if you were an Indian man (*see NNN, I said man, not male*) enrolled as an internal medicine resident, dictated that you would specialize and pursue a fellowship. I trained in an era, sadly, where just like today you were considered an idiot if you stayed a generalist in any field. All of my friends planned to apply for a fellowship, and Patel had told me, "You will specialize. You're too smart to be a general internist." So much pressure, so much confusion—and I wasn't even admitting patients today. I was lost and repeatedly asked anyone and everyone for advice. Somehow the answers were always about lifestyle and money and prestige and respect. Perhaps I was naïve, but I just wanted to learn and help people. Besides, I grew up on a single parent salary of $35K my entire life, and I would make $120K my first year as an internist! This was more money than I had ever imagined. What I didn't understand, but which I appreciate now, is that no one was right or wrong. We just had different value systems and ideas related to opportunity costs, which I had never measured in dollars, although most people did.

Dazed and confused, I decided to join the herd and started to consider a fellowship. Hell, if Patel was going to be a fellow, so would I! Pathetic reasoning, I know. I mused about which field to pursue. Like all other Indian men, I started with cardiology. It was as if all of us had a mutation that somehow forced us to consider a career as a cardiologist. I loved cardiology because I valued the art of the physical exam and loved the idea of evidence-based medicine. The prestige was there. Money was incredible. I would be taking care of the number one killer in America, heart disease. Plenty of uncles were cardiologists, and maybe I could take over their practice (OK, bad idea).

And then I remembered the circadian rhythm and how most heart attacks tend to happen in the early morning hours. No, thanks. I wanted to be Rip Van Winkle for a while to make up for all the missed sleep over the last three years. The clincher? My chairman was a brilliant cardiologist, but he'd slept only five hours a day for the last thirty years! He was always running from one place to another, and although he cared very much, he never seemed to have an opportunity to spend meaningful time consistently with his patients, house staff, and others. I even learned that he was a medical student under NNN! How old was he? We had often talked about how he would have a heart attack from all the exhaustion. He would remind us about the theory of unstable plaques, and what caused them to suddenly rupture. This was his subtle reminder that our less than stellar presentation at the bedside would be the cause of his demise. *At least we would be in the CCU,* I would think silently.

No thank you to cardiology. I handled stress well, but my vision for the future did not involve a beeper going off when I was fifty-five years old, and then running to the ER to take care of an acute MI at 2:30 a.m. Let's see, what about pulmonary and critical care (PCC)? This was an easy out, like the bowler on the Indian cricket team, because PCC rounded on numbers and ventilators, and practiced very little evidence-based medicine—at least in the eye of this misinformed graduating third-year medicine resident. I also liked talking to patients, and how would an intubated patient talk to me? No, thanks.

Infectious disease? Hmmm, interesting. But most of our exposure to the field was in the inpatient setting, where everyone was "septic." We spent all of our time backtracking data related to blood cultures and inappropriate antibiotic use. I think I would have liked infectious disease as a career choice, but I didn't have the desired exposure during residency. No, time to cross it off the list. Rheumatology? Absolutely not! If I see another patient with fibromyalgia, I might develop fibromyalgia by standing next to them. Please! Giving a new name to a patient with a predominantly psychiatric disorder was not for me. I cared, but unfortunately had a habit of not mincing words and always called a spade a spade. Gastroenterology? No thanks, I had been in plenty of GI labs where the fellow would tell the patient that Code Brown (here comes the stool) was natural, and I heard all kinds of sounds coming from an orifice post colonoscopy. Nope, easy elimination; I would not be a stool pigeon. Allergy and immunology? Nah, I'm not much of a bench-top theory research guy. I had done a consult month with Peacock and we had seen just two patients during the entire month. I liked the lifestyle, but this was not for me. Hematology/oncology? It seemed as if it was hard to do one without the other, and this was a field with a specialty within a specialty. You weren't the cancer guy, but the breast cancer guy. You weren't the hematologist, but the leukemia guy. No thanks, I'll pass. Endocrinology? A combination of too much theory and labs with little value on exam skills *(Let's see, I think that thyroid is 27 grams, perhaps 30 grams, but clearly not 35 grams)*, not to mention more outpatient than inpatient experience, eliminated that possibility.

And then a phrase I had heard before hit me: "The only function of the heart is to keep the kidneys alive." Wait a minute! I like numbers, physiology, continuity, a mix of inpatient and outpatient, and I know an uncle in town with a busy practice who actually gave me a stethoscope as a graduation present when I entered medical school. Given such a broad mix of patients, I would still get to practice being a generalist and keep an eye on the heart. Yes, nephrology was it!

I applied for and was excited to land a nephrology fellowship at my institution. I even shared Rockets tickets with a faculty member I called Footloose because he looked like Kevin Bacon. Alas, the marriage with nephrology was over before I knew it. At times, there was need for cross coverage or additional help on the inpatient nephrology service during my residency training. Who should we call? Niraj! He is going to be a fellow anyway, right?

All it took was two months of inpatient nephrology service and I was done. I think I was having fibromyalgia by the end of the first month. I was clinically depressed. I was beyond frustrated with noncompliant patients who missed dialysis appointments and came to the ER as if we were Jiffy Lube. They would receive an oil change and continue to push their engines without an oil change for another ten thousand miles. Please, your car—I mean your body—needs to be here more often even if I use synthetic—I mean prolonged—hemodialysis sessions to get you to your dry weight, or even the fancy KT/V to estimate hemodialysis efficiency. Frankly, I don't even think the renal fellows understood KT/V—and no, I didn't get it either—but it sounded so cool.

Even if patients were compliant with their chronic care follow-up and came to the hospital, their hemodialysis access was clotted or infected. I made phone calls to the surgical service or the infectious disease service every day. Dialysis was supposed to be a bridge towards a more permanent solution known as a transplant, but few patients would be recipients of transplanted kidneys. A greater tragedy? Most patients had progressed to end-stage renal disease requiring hemodialysis because of common controllable diseases like diabetes and hypertension. And yet, if the patients were not compliant in controlling their diabetes and hypertension, why would they be compliant with three-times-a-week dialysis sessions? I realized I loved being a nephrology consultant, but I hated hemodialysis.

I went to see the Chairman of the Department of Nephrology six months before starting my fellowship and stated, "Dr. Bean, I love nephrology, but I hate dialysis."

He had a puzzled look on his face, as if I'd said, "I love French fries, but I hate potatoes." He smiled and responded, "You sound like an internist with an interest in nephrology. Why don't you take a year away from nephrology and see if you miss it?"

I was confused and shocked, but I respected his advice and followed it by taking a detour for a year as an academic internist. My hopes and dreams came true as I became a teacher and a healer at LBJ, never once looking back. Perhaps the road less traveled should be embarked upon more often.

Little did I realize then that my journey and my destination had always been the same: the county hospital known as LBJ.

46

Nirvana

Walkabouts and playground

Residency was full of stories, and the actors, including myself at times, seemed as if they all needed Prozac. Did Prozac come in an aerosolized form? If so, could I convince engineering to put it in the ventilation system? Or perhaps the medication was available in patch form so that it could be delivered at a constant steady state. Unfortunately, no such luck at The County. The party scene was not my thing, and alcohol was but a mistress who guaranteed unforeseen future consequences. Therefore, I tried to find solitude elsewhere. I valued small amounts of quiet time and sanity amid the constant chaos, and I found it in two unlikely sources.

The first source was my walkabouts. Long before my journey to Australia, I would, between seeing patients on call nights or just fifteen minutes before conferences, walk around the hospital parking lot. I would start from one end and walk in a serpentine pattern back and forth through every single lane of the LBJ parking lot. This was my Prozac. It was just me and my thoughts. Somehow in these fifteen minutes, the fog in my head would clear, allowing me to focus. Instead of the constant AMC 26 movies that were simultaneously competing to grab my attention, I could focus on one movie scene at a time. I could see my childhood home in India and friends from my kindergarten class I had not seen in over twenty years. I could be brought to the present moment and focus on the patient I just saw, reflecting on human suffering and why life as a patient seemed so unfair, especially given the limited resources at The County. My unfortunate and unwelcomed companion, the beeper, would always zap me back to reality with the shrill sound of "Wake up, next admission!"

I wondered if I needed an MRI of my brain, an EEG, a psych consult, or all of the above. By the third year of residency, if I was in the hospital and you couldn't find me, everyone would tell you to check the parking lot, my private outback within the fourth largest city in the USA.

If I wasn't in the parking lot, there was only one other place I could be found, and that depended on what time of day you were looking for me. The Internal Medicine Residency Program also had residents who were part of a combined internal medicine and pediatrics residency. I called them TFR (pronounced "tougher") as an oxymoron, since these residents, perhaps from their time spent with kids, were Touchy Feely Residents (TFR). One of them told me that the fourth floor pediatrics area at LBJ actually had a back parallel hallway that led to a rooftop playground. *That's great*, I told myself, *like medicine residents have time for playgrounds. Give me a break, TFR.*

One morning, I actually arrived to the hospital well before NNN's morning report. I think I drove to The County much faster than usual and somehow managed to avoid getting distracted by the fishing show on 610 AM radio. I knew the patients well. Cards were ready. I had a great breakfast, going in the exit door as always. Chest x-rays were accounted for. I still had fifteen minutes but didn't want to chance walkabout and be late. Besides, NNN might see me in the parking lot, and my random self-babbling during a brisk walk might end up being the topic of conversation for the entire morning report. No, thank you. So on a whim, I checked out the so-called playground on the fourth floor. As I opened the door, I thought I had found the gateway to heaven.

This particular side of the hospital faced east. I didn't see the broken portable basketball hoop or the badly worn, outdated play equipment right in front of me. All I could see was the sun rising, and as Depeche Mode suggested, I simply enjoyed the silence. The natural air pollution of Houston only added to the beautiful kaleidoscope of colors that even the Purple Prince from Minneapolis would have been proud of.

This place had been here the whole time and I didn't discover it until my third year of residency? Shut up, Niraj, I told myself. Even the internal voice wasn't going to ruin this glass-half-full moment. Walkabouts and the playground seemed to provide what was consistently missing during my residency: my ability to recognize my own heartbeat. These two outlets gave me a chance to reflect, something that I was not allowed to, much less encouraged to, do during my training. A patient's suffering from a disease was not so different than the angst that all humans, including doctors, go through in this serpentine roller coaster called life. I promised myself then—although I broke the promise many times—that I wouldn't compartmentalize life, for it was all one big HOPESFEARSDREAMSTEARS.

47

Labels

We are but one.

What I'm about to say may not be forgivable, but it needs to be said now as opposed to never: Residency was so busy that I started to take the most important things in life for granted. I neglected to mention to you that after having dealt with my own private serpentine roller coaster, I married my high school sweetheart, Sheila, the love of my life. I know, why didn't I mention this earlier? Like I said, the residency thought process was not always rational.

To continue the theme of "how could you?" it was almost the end of residency in 1996, and my first child was due December 1996. All the pieces of the puzzle entitled HOPESFEARSDREAMSTEARS were starting to take shape, and for the first time, I understood why I was confused. Since my college days, I had used mnemonics as a means to remember everything, and suddenly the puzzle that was me looked like this (see box on next page).

If I were to show this list to my wife, kids, or students, I'm sure that the only thing they would agree on would be the letters *A* and *Z*.

THE NIRAJ PUZZLE FROM A TO Z

Ass

Bright

Conscientious

Dedicated

Egocentric

Father to be

Giving

Hardworking

Irritating

Joker

Kindhearted

Loving

Meandering

Non-negotiating

Obstructive to the status quo

Potty-mouthed

Question-raising

Resentful

Smart

Tough as nails

Undaunted

Victory for truth is all that matters

X-ray vision to see through your bullshit

Your Frenemy

Zen-like confused Indian

I understood why psychiatrists are always in demand. We are all just a bunch of labels overlapping each other, some wanting to be covered up, some wanting to be removed, some placed by others, some perceived by us, some an overestimation, and others a glaring underestimation. In the end, did the labels matter? What are we all chasing in the end, be it patients, doctors, nurses, cafeteria workers, x-ray technicians, friends, families, or enemies? Aren't we all the same? As residency was slowly coming to a close, I again promised myself (and broke the promise many times) that I would be only a label known as HOPESFEARSDREAMSTEARS. I would try to understand others' labels so that in the end, I could better appreciate mine.

48

Guruji

The good versus the bad

The problem with all the bipolarity during residency—in doctors, not patients—was that Zen-like states were few and the Ass-like states were many. We cared but we were exhausted. Our only goal was to somehow find ways to do less work. So we bent the rules to get a sixty- to seventy-hour work week. One resident in particular had mastered the art, and I naturally called him Guruji. Although some of his escapades can never be repeated in print, there were several that I can share with you.

First was the Guruji's brilliance in the MICU. This was arguably the busiest rotation, and with sixteen beds housing complicated patients, sleep was but an unfulfilled dream. We were constantly bombarded with ever-changing information and data points. The Guruji's solution? Make as many patients as possible DNR (Do Not Resuscitate). This was a way of maximizing sleep and minimizing work. The only contraindication to assigning DNR status, according to Guruji, was that the patient was already DNR. Brilliant.

The problem was that I still took my walkabouts and went to the playground. Guruji did not. In my moments of clarity, I would realize that there were issues with Guruji's strategy. Non-intubated patients in their 50s with pneumonia did not require a DNR, especially less than forty-eight hours into their hospital admission. And it got worse. AIDS patients became DNR. Cirrhosis with acute upper GI bleed became DNR. And finally the straw that broke this camel's back: I took care of a DKA (Diabetic Ketoacidosis) patient whom Guruji had made DNR.

"How could you make a DKA patient DNR?" I screamed at Guruji. I had no fear in my eyes or my voice, feeling clearheaded after a walkabout. "I'm a diabetic, too!"

"Then perhaps you should be DNR," he responded. "In fact, I think that the ketones I smell on your breath are clouding your judgment," he went on.

"It's the damn Tic Tac, you moron!" I retorted.

"Interesting. What flavor?" he asked.

I was a fuming brown man turning into shades of my favorite coffee. *And to think we all considered you our role model. You suck!*

There were three upper-level residents in the MICU, each responsible for overnight call every 3 days. Given the Guruji's need to make every patient DNR, a daily clarification was needed for each one's code status. How could someone who was DNR twenty-four hours earlier now suddenly be considered a full code patient? You can imagine the tension, confusion—and years later, the laughter. We never told on residents during training. At the time, we had an us-against-the-world mentality. It is only now that I realize the consequences of blindly worshipping Gurujis. Marx was correct. Religion is indeed the opium of the masses. Labels are never healthy, except maybe HOPESFEARSDREAMSTEARS.

The other strategy that Guruji had towards the sixty- to seventy-hour work week dream was how to show everyone he was busy even if he wasn't. The best example was one morning report with NNN. Patel had already been excused for Diwali (though I knew that slacker was teeing up to play golf), so it was just Guruji presenting the patients. NNN looked at the cards and had his usual "that's interesting" look on his face. Guruji started, "Good morning, oh worthy, oh great, oh omnipotent NNN. I hope you will be merciful and kind this morning because Patel is not here and I'm just exhausted, completely exhausted, your highness, from a ton of patients I admitted last night."

I'm exaggerating the obsequiousness, but I already felt nauseous, and I wasn't even on my third cup of coffee yet. NNN looked at the cards and retorted, "You say that you admitted a ton of patients. Did I hear you correctly?"

"Yes," responded Guruji.

"That's not possible" said NNN. "I only have three cards here. Did you just admit three new patients or are you just lazy and didn't turn in the rest of the cards?"

I was feeling better already. Guruji was about to get his ass kicked. *An instant panacea for nausea,* I thought, smirking out of the side of my transient Bell's palsy mouth. "No, sir, your greatness," responded Guruji. "You're right as always related to the number of patients I admitted. It is three. I admitted three new patients and thus per your request turned in three cards."

NNN was troubled. "You say you turned in three cards on three new patients and yet you are exhausted from having admitted a ton of patients? Please explain to the group how that is possible."

Guruji dryly responded. "NNN, the combined weight of the three patients was over 2,000 pounds, and thus as you can see, I admitted a ton of patients and am exhausted from thinking about the sheer—how should I put this delicately without lack of respect to my patients—the sheer weight of the problem."

NNN burst out laughing, and thank God for that, because the rest of us were not too far behind. Guruji was a smart ass like me, but unlike me he already understood that the art of medicine went well beyond Harrison's *Principles of Internal Medicine*. The best panacea for any tense situation was laughter, the best medicine.

Morning report ended early that day, and for a smidgen of our residency, there was no fear. Just like all other events throughout my residency, I was reminded of *A Tale of Two Cities*; "It was the best of times, it was the worst of times." I hoped that before it was too late, as the book suggested, wisdom was around the corner.

49

It's Finally Over

Saying goodbye is the hardest thing.

It was the last day of residency, and I had completed the required checklist, which included turning in your call room keys, badge, beeper, and parking card, amongst other essentials that were really nonessential in the grand scheme of things. I still had work to do, though. I had asked The County if they would hire me directly to work at LBJ, but was told that there was no precedent for such action. Disappointed, I signed on to stay with academia but would start at the Hermann Hospital/Clinic, hoping I could eventually get back full-time to LBJ.

Given what I considered to be a temporary detour, I had to say goodbye. It started with a cup of coffee and a sunrise as I sat on the slide in the playground, a gentle tear forming in my eye. For a surreal moment, it seemed as if someone's hand wiped away the tear, but there was no one there but my memories. The next stop was breakfast at the cafeteria. My surprise? The breakfast tray was already there for me when I arrived. I had tears in my eyes, and without saying a word I went back out and for the first time came in through the entrance door. After a hug that seemed, like

Willie Nelson's song, a "moment of forever" with my Nazi cafeteria friend, I was off to the next stop on memory lane.

I went out the exit door for a change, and around the corner was the radiology reading room. More hugs to remind me that we were anything but the skeletal images I had taken for granted for the last three years. Then I took a walk up through 3C, 3B, 3A, 4C, and 4B. Habits were hard to break, and this was the order I'd always done my rounds with the team. More hugs, which were nothing more than HOPESFEARSDREAMSTEARS. I had already said goodbye to my clinic patients and nurses earlier in the week. I had just one more stop to make.

I knocked on NNN's office door. I could hear the shuffling as he slowly moved away from his desk. "Oh, hello, Niraj. Come in. Everything alright?"

I already had a lump in my throat, and I guess he must have seen the look in my eyes. *Such an observant clinician, NNN,* I thought.

"No, everything is fine. It's just that I have a confession to make. As you know, today is my last day of residency, and well, I don't know a damn thing. It's not just syphilis that is the great imitator. Hell, the entire field of medicine is a great imitator, and I'm confused. The whole field is gray. Why can't there be some crystal-clear black or white area in what we do?

"NNN, I'm scared that I'm going to hurt people," I replied.

He listened. He was always an amazing listener. He pulled up a chair for me and told me something I will never forget. "Niraj, congratulations, you've finally become a doctor. My job here is done with you. You finally understand that asking questions that lead to more questions and at times confusion is, in essence, the art of our profession. It is the pompous arrogant assholes who think they know everything but have no time for self- reflection and no time for communicating with their patients that I worry about. You're an asshole, but a good one. Yes, I know about your walkabouts, but don't worry, your secret is safe with me. Why do you think I run so much?

"I wish you the best, but do me a favor and spread the gospel in the future. The journey is shorter than you think. Look at me, I'm a fossil, and someday you will be too. I'm proud to call you my clone and take pride when I hear you've pissed someone off for the right reasons. Hell, someone the other day told me I had created a monster, and I knew it had to be you!"

I was SpongeBob, weepy beyond repair by now, but I had a gift for him that I had brought back from India. It was a statue of elephants following one another, trunk to tail, in a circle. He had told the residents, including me, more than once that we were a bunch of elephants following each other around in circles, not knowing who was leading whom and why, with the tragedy that in the end, we were right back where we started.

He told me this was the second-best present he had ever received from a resident, the first being the toilet paper roll distinguishing you-know-what from shinola. The story took him fifteen minutes, but for that moment he was thirty years younger, and there was a gleam in his eyes. I patiently let him finish the story I already knew, because even this selfish resident had finally learned that not everything revolved around me. I understood that residency and life were one and the same, and where as one had just ended, the other was just beginning. Maybe Sharukh Khan was right in *Om Shanti Om*. In all moments of sadness, no one needs to worry, because life is like a Hindi movie and "Picture abhi baaki hei mere dost." HOPESFEARSDREAMSTEARS.

ACT III

The Attending Years

Age of Wisdom

"Knowledge speaks, but wisdom listens."

Jimmy Hendrix

50

The Beginning

Square peg, round hole

It started as a medical student and continued through residency, my seemingly unending search to find a place where I belonged. Now that I was an attending, still too young to be called a pretending by the residents, it was no different. There was no point in trying to fit a square peg into a round hole. There was no right or wrong. Different people have different value systems, and as an extension different HOPESFEARSDREAMSTEARS.

I started out my academic career as a "Clinical Instructor." I think this was a way for the department chairman to make sure Jim Adler, the tough, smart lawyer known as the Texas Hammer, was not coming to say goodbye to a promising young career with another lawsuit. Since The County was not hiring, I started working in the medical center, hoping eventually to return to my heart and soul: LBJ.

On the surface, I had everything one might wish for: A fancy corner office in a historic building with floor to ceiling windows and 180-degree views of Rice University and downtown Houston. A $120K salary, which was approximately four times more than my dad earned and clearly more than I had ever dreamed of making. Everyone was always smiling and cordial. I even spent some time in the fancy university hospital across the street as the attending on a teaching service, trying to provide a fine balance between inpatient and outpatient medicine.

But something was clearly missing. On the inpatient service at a semi-private hospital, we were "encouraged" to call consult services for "educational purposes." What was my role, then, as an educator in encouraging residents to learn by asking questions and fostering a conversation towards a lifelong journey? A quote from Hemingway's *Death in an Afternoon* came to mind: "If we are to converse about a bullfight, I must assume you have been to one." How could residents learn if all they did was call seven consults on every patient? How could they respectfully agree to disagree and challenge the consult service if the residents did not independently read about the bullfight?

I had trained under the NNN old-school regime and was thus reminded of another quote from Shakespeare: "Let every eye negotiate itself and trust no agent." I believed in the team concept, but was taught to question everything and trust myself without making assumptions based on information provided by others. Working in the medical center provided very little opportunity for academic stimulation, especially for a general internist like me. Every note became a "have to," not a "want to," and served the singular purpose of billing at the highest level possible. Sadly, my addendums to the daily resident notes began to mirror those of my colleagues: "Agree with above."

I was becoming the pretending that I had despised during my training, the one I'd promised myself that I would never become. I had a beautiful wife, a daughter on the way, great working hours, money, and parents who constantly bragged about their doctor son. However, I was unhappy and bleedingHOPESFEARSDREAMSTEARS. Something needed to change before I no longer recognized the man in the mirror. This had become a race to see if either the reflection or the mirror would crack first.

How could I get back to my beloved LBJ? Actually, it was easier than I thought. Not surprisingly, one's academic promotion was linked to visibility. As such, LBJ was viewed by most academic physicians as Cinderella, an albatross that would only limit their advancement. The Department of General Internal Medicine did not have a single faculty member that was full-time at LBJ. It was not the department's fault. What I didn't understand at this young, idealistic age was that at the beginning, middle, end, top, bottom, side, width, length, depth, and any other measurement you could come up with, money makes the world go around. The department simply could not afford to place a full-time faculty member at LBJ.

But what about things that are unmeasured? How do you measure making a difference in the life of an indigent patient who was just like you and I but wore a mask called poverty, a mask that could not be removed? After all, during the holidays, why do most of us donate to charity? I simply wanted to donate my time, my life, and my career to a place that had somehow changed me for the better. It was not a holier-than-thou impulse. It wasn't right or wrong. It was just me being me, nothing more and nothing less. I knew where I belonged, and more importantly, where I stuck out like a sore thumb.

So, why was making my way back to The County easier than I thought? No one wanted to be at The County as a faculty member. This was clearly in my favor. Slowly but surely I would ask faculty members if they wanted to trade a month of inpatient service at LBJ for a month of inpatient service at the fancy medical center hospital, which was separated from the medical school by a two-way driveway. Visibility, remember? It seemed like a trick question given the verbal and nonverbal clues I noticed when I asked the question. "Are you joking?" "Are you serious?" "What else do you want in return?" "Have you checked your thyroid function tests lately because you must be headed towards myxedema coma?" The nonverbal clues were just as hilarious. Eyebrows that would have put Mr. Spock to shame would rise asymmetrically. Fascinating indeed. A transient unintended Bell's palsy was also common as were horizontal tonic neck movements indicating utter disbelief.

My transition back to The County would require baby steps, but I was beginning to crawl. It started with two to three months of inpatient service trades my first year and grew from there. Kojak (the name I gave my boss, for obvious reasons) was also supportive. After all, he was politically shrewd—an inherent trait that over the years must have cost him all of his hair—and understood who didn't belong in the medical center.

Within three years of finishing my residency, I was back at LBJ full-time. HOPESFEARSDREAMSTEARS came true! Now that I had created a new word that could be separated into parts but seemed to belong together, I too became one with The County in my heart, in my mind, and in my soul.

51

Intentions

Lacking political shrewdness to understand perceptions

I had always reminded myself that I wouldn't be like other pretendings. If you ask medical students or residents, they will tell you that clinical education is especially frustrating during medical school. The following quote, equally humorous and tragic, summarizes one's journey during training: "Experience is what allows one to make the same mistakes over and over again with a higher level of confidence." In fact, I used to chuckle every time our pretending would start yet another educational conversation with "In my experience…"

Everyone learned on their own. I believed in autonomy, but independence without appropriate evidence-based supervision is lethal. I knew this better than most, having hurt patients physically and emotionally during residency. We weren't baking cakes. One can always try again if the cake doesn't turn out as intended. But we were trying to save lives—or at least alter morbidity if we couldn't alter mortality. During our undergraduate years, I suspect that regardless of the generational shift in educational attitudes or the career pathway that we chose, all of us had a systematic way of learning. Somewhere along the way there was a manual, a textbook, or a syllabus. No such system of learning seemed to exist during medical school or residency. Perhaps there were too many parallel competing systems that were driven by experience without objective evidence.

I don't remember once being asked an open-ended question such as "How would you change your medical school or residency training?" Lectures were haphazard. Rounds were rushed. At times, I wasn't even sure how many of our teachers were actually qualified to be teachers, including myself. Did we have any formal training? No. Did most pretendings want to teach? No. Why? Teaching, as I would find out years later, was the slowest route to promotion in academic medicine, although for me it was the most rewarding. Early in my career, I was told that hanging out with medical students and residents (teaching) and providing direct care to patients was a "have to, not a want to." "Don't worry," said the Ivory Tower Gods, "once you start getting grants, you can do inpatient service just one month every year." *But what if I actually like teaching?* I would ask myself silently during sessions with my bosses.

No, I wasn't going to become a pretending. Or at least, I tried very hard not to put on a mask that in time I would no longer be able to remove. Unfortunately, there were consequences of taking such a hard stance: I was a fish out of water. My rounds, and by extension my hospital teaching service, were extremely busy and demanding. I use the term "unfortunately" because as a naïve young attending, I believed in intention. I cared and wanted to make my learners better by teaching each individual and taking care of one patient at a time in a non-hurried format. Sadly, my bosses only believed in perception. *Who is he to ask so many questions of everything that everyone is doing? We've always done it this way.*

And just like perceptions of primary care in general, I

was being crucified behind closed doors for the *N* of 1 patient who allegedly had a poor outcome due to my actions. What about the N of 99 that did well on my service? It was not relevant if I practiced cost-effective medicine, or if my patients had the shortest length of stay or lowest readmission rates. Instead, what one saw was the questioning of the status quo. No one bothered to ask me directly about the *N* of 1, and as such I had erroneously assumed all was well. After all, no doctor has ever had a batting average of 1.000, and I believed that failures were crucial for future successes. I was taught by NNN that if I had a 100% approval rating, perhaps I wasn't doing my job. Sadly, I failed to recognize that such thoughts were only allowed by those in the field with gray hair or frankly without any hair at all. At that time, however, unbeknownst to me, I was not a member of the Hair Club for Men.

No one was right and no one was wrong. The leadership and I were cut from a different cloth. I was all about intention. My bosses were all about perception. I wish I knew then what I know now, having completed a recent Master Teacher's Fellowship, which included lectures on disagreements in the workplace and conflict resolution.

Sadly, my HOPESFEARSDREAMSTEARS did not match those of others. Square peg Niraj belonged at The County, just not at The County that was still governed by bosses who fit into round holes.

52

Rounds

Commandments, cards, and beyond

My team was on call every fourth day, similar to my training during medical school and residency. What one knows, one sees. With an understanding of what I liked and disliked— based on experience at the time because no one had mentored me on evidence-based education yet—I modeled my rounds on NNN's Socratic method of asking questions. Like NNN, I had high expectations, and my own Ten Commandments (see next page).

The structure for post-call rounds was the same. Each student, intern, and resident would make out an NNN card. I had discussed the format and expectations in detail with each team at the start of the rotation. However, unlike the NNN card, I would give each card one of three possible faces: a smiley face, a neutral face—I had to keep emphasizing it was neutral since it looked like a frowny face at first glance—and a frowny face. If you earned a smiley face, I kept the card because it represented a job well done. If you received a neutral face or a frown, you would need to revise the findings on the back of the card and then resubmit it. If it was accepted, you were awarded a smiley face. If not, you would get another neutral or frowny face on the back of the card, and

ATTENDING ROUNDS COMMANDMENTS

1) Thou shall not make excuses.

2) Thou shall not be lazy, and lying will not be tolerated. Do not bullshit physical exams.

3) Thou shall always be on time for rounds, which will be at 6:00 a.m. on post-call days and at 9:15 a.m. on non-post-call days.

4) Thou shall know details on each patient. No exceptions are made, even if you are just covering the patient for the day because your colleague is off (see rule # 1).

5) Thou shall be ready to defend every action you took on rounds using medical evidence, not just experience. Don't order tests without a reason.

6) Thou shall understand that the correct answer isn't "I don't know." It is "I don't know, but I'll find out."

7) Thou shall understand Lobe's Laws of Medicine:

   Rule # 1: If what you're doing is working, keep on doing it.
   Rule # 2: If what you're doing isn't working, stop doing it.
   Rule # 3: If you don't know what to do, don't do anything.
   Rule # 4 (some might say the most important rule): Never let a surgeon touch your patient unless it's a matter of life or death.

8) Thou shall understand "If we are to converse about a bullfight, I must assume you have been to one." Ernest Hemingway's *Death in the Afternoon*: The idea being that you can't have an intelligent conversation with other colleagues unless you understand the topic of the conversation. If you're asking for an opinion from Cardiology on a patient with congestive heart failure, make sure you understand congestive heart failure. Do not assume that Cardiology is always right and you're always wrong.

9) Thou shall understand "Let every eye negotiate for itself and trust no agent." William Shakespeare's *Much Ado about Nothing*: Don't blindly follow recommendations made by anyone, including your current pretending (me), and always look for objective data to confirm "he said, she said" subjective perceptions.

10) Thou shall understand the CARD designed by NNN and use it to guide your thought process.

it would be returned to you for more corrections. The process would not end until you achieved a smiley face. The goal wasn't to torture you, but to get you to understand that I would be engaged in your educational journey and wouldn't be satisfied until you understood the errors involved in your thought process.

Discussion was encouraged, and everyone was allowed to challenge and question one other, including their pretending. The goal was to get at least seventy-five percent of the cards to identify the correct problem within the first two attempts by the end of the rotation. Given my high demands and expectations, there was much heart rate variability during my rotation. Ah, I was helping my learners live longer without realizing it.

My rounds started at 6:00 a.m. and wouldn't stop for external forces. I would continue with the students and interns even after the upper-level residents left for NNN, whose morning report had been moved to 7:30 a.m. There was always pin-drop silence when I entered the radiology reading area at 5:55 a.m. To start the day, I would ask for the chief complaint on each new admission. As usual, I got the "I'm a resident, what the hell does it matter? Let's just cut to the chase!" version. For example, the upper-level resident would note that the chief complaint was congestive heart failure. Such shortcuts would accelerate my own heart rate independent of the can of Diet Coke, The County's breakfast of champions that was always in my hand along with the Tic Tac in my mouth.

I taught by asking questions, and thus began the educational journey. "Did you not learn in medical school that the chief complaint is stated in the patient's own words, and reflects why they came to the hospital? Let me give you an example. You say congestive heart failure. First of all, let's assume that you have the correct problem—not the diagnosis, mind you, just the problem—but we'll come to that later. Do you think that if the chief complaint was as follows 'problemas con mi resparacion,' meaning 'I have problems with my breathing,' that perhaps you would get some insight into the fact there is a language barrier and how it may impact care both during the admission and subsequent follow-up. If you had such information, do you think that if given a choice as a patient that he or she might want to have a resident who was fluent in Spanish taking care of him or her? How many of you have ever scheduled a patient for follow-up with an effort to make sure the doctor they would be seeing could also speak the same language, most importantly here at LBJ, Spanish?"

There were no raised hands and all eyes were fixed to the floor. "I know you're probably thinking, 'but Dr. Mehta, my patient speaks English.' Ok, what if the chief complaint was, again assuming this is congestive heart failure, 'Doc, I can't move the boxes at work anymore.' Would that generate some more questions that you should be asking related to his work? What kind of work? Is this occupational lung disease mimicking congestive heart failure? Is this person lifting boxes at a shipyard, and if so, is this a mechanical back problem or something more sinister? If he isn't able to work, is he alone or does he provide for others as the breadwinner in the family? If he can't work, how will he pay for his medicines? In order to take care of patients, you must be patient, and in order to provide care, you must first care."

I would receive one of two responses in the form of nonverbal clues, especially since I had great peripheral vision and eyes in the back of my head. *(No, Mom and Dad, slow down your heart rate. I'm not a demigod.)* The responses? "You're an asshole and I can't wait for this rotation to end" or "You're an asshole, but I'm willing to give you a chance to prove you're an asshole who cares."

This was just the chief complaint, and our discussion

took the amount of time it took most pretendings to complete rounds on one patient. I applied the same theory in teaching the learner regardless of his or her level of training and refused to be deterred by bad attitude, especially since I had been the poster child at one time of all that I was seeing. What came after the chief complaint in the journey of education that I hoped was equal parts art and science? The first set of vital signs recorded when the patient came to the emergency room. This would also lead to more questions. What is the function of vital signs? What are the characteristics of vital signs that make them so useful? Do you think based on these vital signs that this patient is stable or headed for rapid decompensation? Why did three of you say yes and five of you say no to the last question? If you disagree, do you know why? What is a kappa value and what does it measure?

By now, I think their opinions had changed from two possibilities to a single consensus answer: "Asshole!" I really did care, but hoped they would understand the value of tough love. As my colleagues would say over the years, "Damn it, Niraj, you have the demands of a surgeon on a medical service, and you're an asshole just like them. Maybe you should've been a surgeon!" Being an internist, I could never tell if I was being complimented or insulted every time I was called a surgeon personality, Type A Personality, or Asshole. It did not help that I even had an earlobe crease, known as Frank's Sign, which is purportedly associated with such personality traits.

Each vital sign would raise more questions, from pulse pressure to fever-pulse deficit to the classic LBJ-specific vital sign: respiratory rate. Since I started medical school in 1989, it seemed as if every single patient at LBJ was breathing at twenty times a minute. Doctors, nurses, and even medical students knew that this was not normal. Although variations in respiratory rate were dependent on an individual patient's age, time of day, and underlying medical conditions, twenty times a minute was absurd. And thus, at LBJ anything other than twenty times a minute meant something was wrong or that you were lucky enough to have a diligent nurse. Although it was usually the latter, to humor myself, I always assumed it was the former, since a diligent nurse was deemed an oxymoron. If you used the term "diligent nurse" as a doctor, you would be ostracized for suggesting such a person existed. I learned later that they did exist, and I could never have become the physician I always wished to be without help from the nursing staff.

Having discussed the patient's chief complaint and vital signs, I shifted the educational focus to the chest x-ray. What was the most important thing about the chest x-ray? The answer: a previous x-ray for comparison, since we were Eternal Medicine and needed to see dynamic changes. Puzzled glances would require further explanation. For example, I would ask if a patient smokes, has lost weight, and has a right upper lobe mass on the chest x-ray, what would you think about? Even my myxedematous medical student would chime in, "lung cancer."

Brownnoser, another student would be thinking. *Gunner* would be the thought from yet a third. Interns were thinking, *Asshole, he wasn't asking you. You're making me look bad.* The resident was thinking, *I'm getting my ass kicked before NNN! Who the hell does this guy think he is, NNN Jr?*

"Yes, excellent, but what if I showed you a chest x-ray from seven years ago that had the exact same mass lesion with no change? Would you still think this patient had lung cancer?"

"No" would be the answer from three people now.

"Why not?" I would ask.

"Because tumors have doubling time," would respond the intern, beating out the gunner who was slow on the

Jeopardy response button.

"Excellent. So, if the answer is no, does that change your likelihood of other possibilities? Could weight loss be a manifestation of other disease processes in addition to cancer? If so, is the cause metabolic, congenital, infectious, vascular, or autoimmune in origin? Perhaps, the weight loss is a manifestation of a weakened immune system or maybe your patient is homeless and doesn't have the privilege of eating three times a day like all of us. Maybe due to circumstances beyond your patient's control, weight loss is a manifestation of substance abuse or depression. And finally, perhaps the chest x-ray abnormality is an incidentaloma, and unrelated to the weight loss."

Slowly, I could see the twinkle in the eyes of at least a couple of learners. Eureka! The rest were still thinking *asshole,* but at least somewhere in the room there was HOPESFEARSDREAMSTEARS. "We will learn together, and I will try very hard not to be your pretending, and you in turn will try very hard to stop pretending you know everything."

Having finished my holy trinity of chief complaint, vital signs, and chest x-ray, it was time to move teaching to the bedside. I would start with new patients admitted in the emergency room followed by 3C, 3B, 3A, 4C, and 4B. Bedside rounds would end on 3D-MICU if we had a patient awaiting transfer, but "bed was being cleaned" on the general wards. Usually this meant the patient who had vacated the bed was going home or to the big home in the sky. I was old school and took Osler's quote to heart: "He who studies medicine without books sails an uncharted sea, but he who studies medicine without patients does not go to sea at all." I was so tired of training under multiple pretendings who did so-called table rounds ("agree with above" notes on chart) or barely touched patients—much less communicated their thoughts to family members—that I had vowed to spend as much time at the bedside as possible.

Perhaps Osler wasn't entirely correct, since technically even pretendings were "seeing" patients, believing a handshake and an "agree with above" note justified billing for services provided. I would paraphrase Osler and suggest that "rounding without examining and spending time with patients and family members is like booking daily vacations on the Titanic." I had personally hit plenty of icebergs during my training but now found myself captain of the ship. I finally hoped to guide the ship in the right direction by providing autonomy guided by supervision.

This was the toughest act for any teaching attending. Since there were four patients per room at LBJ, I would start the discussion outside the room to provide some degree of privacy. The team would place the charts for all patients in a small cart with dividers. This was important because at times I would want confirmatory evidence during rounds. I also wanted to use the card system, having hated the on average eighty-hour work week during residency. By using the cards, I hoped to provide a fine balance between proficiency and efficiency so the team could get home at a reasonable hour.

No one liked change, and as such the first week of rounding on the post-call day was the most difficult. My wife, Sheila, used to joke that I should take an alternate route home so that my learners would not attempt to run me off the road. It seemed as if few attendings asked questions, paid close attention to physical exam findings, or demanded evidence for actions taken by residents. As a result, rounds were usually two hours long, regardless of the number of admissions. Let's do some math. Our maximum number of new admissions, established after I finished residency, was sixteen patients. Two hours = 120 minutes. So, the pretending would be seeing on average one patient every seven-and-a-half minutes! This would include a presentation of the history and physical exam, bedside confirmation and teaching of interesting physical exam findings, and communication of the attending's thoughts of the likely diagnosis, plan of action, expected duration of hospital stay, and future plans for outpatient follow-up to the patient and the patient's caregivers. Even if the pretending ran like Usain Bolt, he wouldn't win the race. Oh, and the seven-and-a-half minutes did not account for travel time for patients located on different units. Did I mention that on average, each team also had eight previous patients who perhaps had issues overnight and required further assistance or guidance?

A hundred and twenty minutes, my ass! There was no wrong or right, and I was not holier-than-thou. My value system was different and I simply wasn't going to use the same excuse I had heard over and over again: "The system is broken and it's impossible to fix it. Besides, this is how I learned, and residents need to learn the same way."

"Really? And did you like your training?" I'd counter.

"No, I hated it!"

"Well, then why don't you do something about it?"

"Because my boss doesn't care if I round for two hours or six hours. Besides I have grant papers to write."

"Doesn't it matter to you? Doesn't it matter to your patients? Do you think your patients could pick you out of a lineup as the attending of record responsible for their care? Or should I just be blunt and ask you if you could pick the patient out of a lineup since you did 'table rounds.'"

I wanted to be the change I wished to see, as Gandhiji had suggested over fifty years ago. It was sad, but the care a patient received during training was only as good as the one provided by the lead resident or fellow, and I panned to change that. I hoped that students, residents, and eventually my colleagues would understand that there was no "I" in team. We were on this journey together and needed to learn from each other's fears. In sharing the important task of helping acutely ill patients, I dreamed that although the journey was long, it would serve as our destination because we would travel together to wipe away each other's tears. Alas, my idealism made me the lone ranger in a movie no one else wanted to star in.

Rounds would continue, using the card method, outside each room. Why? It was the simplest way to balance proficiency and efficiency while allowing for the Socratic method of teaching. Here is the traditional method of presenting the entire history and physical exam on every new patient. Keep in mind that it was not only possible but likely that you would have sixteen new admissions every fourth day on call.

Student: "Patient is a fifty-seven-year-old woman who is here with chest pain. The chest pain started yesterday afternoon while the patient was watching Oprah. It felt like a mild heartburn and she had read in a magazine before that apple juice could help heartburn. So, the patient decided to drink apple juice and the pain went away for few minutes. It came back again and she wasn't sure what to do. So she called Aunt Angina who told her that soda water could help her burp it out. She tried to drink some Coca-Cola, but it didn't help. Oprah was finished so she decided to take her usual afternoon nap, but awoke again with chest pain at 6:00 p.m. She knew it was 6:00 p.m. because the evening news was just starting. Her left arm was tingling a little now and she was a bit worried. She denies shortness of breath, nausea, vomiting, dizziness, palpitations, constipation, diarrhea, abdominal pain, blurry vision, presyncopal symptoms, or anything like that. She has never had anything like this happen before. Dad died of heart attack when he was fifty-two years old, and mom had diabetes. She took all of her evening medicines and ate a little bit, thinking the pain would go away. It stayed past the news hour and she called her daughter, who told her to call 911. So, she came to our emergency room. Her past vaccines are all updated except for tetanus. Her surgical history is important for gallbladder removal twenty-seven years ago, and I confirmed it, she has a gallbladder surgery scar. Socially she smokes one pack per day of cigarettes but is trying to cut down and denies alcohol or IV drug abuse. Her review of system shows a four-pound weight loss over last three months, on/off joint pain, seasonal congestion attributed to allergies, and sometimes she can't sleep through the night because she thinks she worries too much about her daughter. She has no allergies. Her past medical history includes diabetes, hypertension, fatigue, depression, arthritis, and irritable bowel syndrome. She was told she may be hypothyroid before but is not sure and is not taking any medications although someone told her she could have a goiter. Her current medications include metformin, hydrochlorothiazide, lisinopril, Bentyl, Motrin, and Cymbalta. She doesn't know the dosage and didn't bring her medications."

This was just the history. The presenter had not even described the physical exam, reported the lab values, or shared other relevant data such as the EKG or chest x-ray. Half the team was already wishing they were somewhere else. The other half was already there. The attention span for any attending is about five minutes, which is perfect, I guess since we only had seven-and-a-half minutes per patient. And with a presentation like the one above, the attending was already having acute delayed DTRs (deep tendon reflexes) from progressing to myxedema coma! Ah, but the card could change that. The same patient would be presented as follows:

Problem: Unstable Angina
Diagnosis: Coronary Artery Disease

I would ask my student about the evidence for unstable angina. Instead of the timeline of Oprah and the evening news, a better answer might be, "increasing levels of chest pain with recurrence at rest or with lesser levels of activity." "I don't know" was sometimes the answer. If so, I could involve other members of the team, again by asking the question, "what is unstable angina?" Each question in turn could lead to additional questions such as

1) What is the treatment for unstable angina?
2) How do you know this is not Prinzmetal's angina?
3) Could this be cocaine-induced chest pain?
4) What changes do you see on an EKG for unstable angina?

Each one of these questions could open a subset of questions, and depending on the level of the learner—student, intern, or resident—I could lead a discussion by asking more sophisticated questions focusing not only on diagnosis and treatment, but also involving prognosis and harm.

This was just the beginning. If the answer for evidence of unstable angina was "new onset congestive heart failure in setting of chest pain," I could move the conversation to congestive heart failure. I might ask an open-ended question such as "What is your evidence for congestive heart failure?" The student might say, "I think I heard an S3." I could ask, "What is an S3?" and ask the differential of other sounds in early diastole, such as an opening snap, a tumor plop, a pericardial knock, or an S2 split.

"What causes these other sounds and can one distinguish them at the bedside?" I'd query. Then I'd ask the student to tap the sound on the wall. Finally, I would ask the student to tap an S4 to see if he or she could distinguish the two sounds. "Could you do this if the heart rate was elevated? If not, could you slow down the heart rate, and if so how?"

By now, the intern might chime in and ask about crackles on the lung exam. The resident might suggest that the chest x-ray showed pulmonary edema. I was now able to generate an active conversation, which would eventually lead to what I called the "I wonder" moment. When this happened, I knew that I had finally gotten through to the learner, and created a lifelong bond related to education. To this day, NNN and I share such an unbreakable bond based on mutual trust and respect.

In this case, an intern actually paused and asked the question: "Dr. Mehta, I wonder which one of these is actually the best test to rule in or rule out congestive heart failure?"

"Excellent question, Patel." Interestingly, the number of Patels in medical school never decreases. "I assume like all other Patel internal medicine residents that you are also considering cardiology?"

"Yes, Dr. Mehta, how did you know?"

"People used to think I was Patel, but since that is a story for another day, let's just say I have the rare Indian mutation that precluded me from pursuing a career in cardiology."

Chuckles and half-smiles would follow.

"Why don't we all go home tonight and try to find an answer to that question, and that includes me," I'd suggest.

Our conversation about the evidence supporting the diagnosis would continue. Unlike NNN's morning report, however, I had the actual chart, and more importantly, the physical exam. We would now enter the room, and meet the patient and his or her family members. If you didn't see a family member at LBJ, something was wrong. Actually, if you saw fewer than five family members at LBJ, something was wrong. I would explain to the patient that I would be asking personal questions, examining them, and teaching the students and residents. To reassure them, I made it clear that I would finish with an explanation of our plan and time to answer any questions. I would also remind them that I appreciated their cooperation especially with a large group of learners. I encouraged them to stop me at any point if I made them feel uncomfortable. I would establish rapport by gently holding the patient's hand and maintaining eye contact. Once trust was established, I focused on the power of observation: what we know, we see. As such, the Socratic Method continued at the bedside but only after I reminded the team to pull the curtain for privacy. I would also instruct the team to ask other patients in the room to respectfully turn down the television volume for a few minutes.

"So, what do you see?" was always the opening question. I still haven't figured out why learners think that looking at other parts of the room will save them from answering the question. I would start with an open-ended question without directing it towards a particular team member. Why? I wanted to know who was curious, who was shy, who was quick to answer, who was afraid, and who wasn't interested. I also didn't want anyone to think I was picking on them. As I became comfortable with the team, and more importantly when they understood my intentions, I could direct questions to a specific member.

Since there was always a predictable silence early on during the rotation, I would repeat the question, "Again, so what do you see?" At times, the patient would break the tension by answering, "I see a lot of confused doctors." Nervous chuckles would follow. If I didn't get a volunteer, I would go around the room and ask each member the question.

Typical answers on patients such as the one we were discussing would be. . . .

Student Gunner: "I see a patient who is lying at a 60 degree angle probably to relieve the elevated filling pressure due to his congestive heart failure."

Student Shy: "I, um, I see mild distress but otherwise patient seems comfortable."

Student I'm Not Going into Medicine: "I don't know what I see." (Silently)

Student Brown Noser: "Dr. Mehta, I respectfully agree with the wonderful observations made by my colleagues and I would also like to respectfully add that perhaps his neck veins are distended but then again I don't have the level of expertise as the rest of the team and may be wrong."

Categorical Medicine Intern (meaning doing three years of internal medicine training): "He is mildly short of breath and has an IV pole with medication which is Lasix since I ordered it."

Preliminary Intern (meaning maximum of one year internal medicine as a "have to not a want to," usually counting days towards something else including, but not limited to dermatology or anesthesiology). This was the trickiest because there was usually no middle ground with preliminary interns. They were either brilliant or might as well have been

Dr. "I'm Not Going Into Medicine." This particular one was not interested and responded: "Ditto."

Resident I'm Staying General: "He is comfortable, has good color, and I don't see any cyanosis."

Resident I'm Going into Cardiology, aka Patel: "Well, I see many things. For starters, I noticed that the oxygen that he is supposed to get via nasal cannula is actually oxygenating his bed which doesn't look cyanotic to me *(What a smart ass, I thought. I think we will get along just fine)*. He also has Cheyne-Stokes respiration, which is a predictor of poor outcome in congestive heart failure. His neck veins are distended, but I do not see Kussmaul neck veins with engorgement during inspiration decreasing the likelihood of a constrictive or restrictive cardiomyopathy."

Patient in Question: "I like your accent."

Thank God we were temporarily saved from further observations by Patel's DOTM (Diarrhea Of The Mouth). It was now my turn.

"First of all, excellent observations. Remember, there is no wrong or right answer and we're just having a conversation to learn from one another. I see a middle-aged man who is surrounded by family members, suggesting he has a great support system. There is food from home meaning he won't die of eating hospital food." Humor was my greatest asset; after all, it had helped me survive medical school and residency.

"He has a Bible on the table next to him and he either likes watching game shows (*The Price is Right* was on with the volume turned down) or the TV is just a distraction. I want to make sure in time I teach you to heal with equal parts heart and mind. I want you to think like a human being first and like a doctor second. Since you will appreciate some of the principles of medicine as you get older, but still need a way to card catalogue massive amount of information that you are taught as pearls, I will try to simplify your learning by providing you mnemonics for almost everything. Since first impressions are important, as a young doctor to be or in training, here is your mnemonic for the day related to observations as you walk into the room" (see box on next page).

My intention was always the same: I just wanted to teach and lead by example. This wasn't about me trying to impress anyone. I had always hoped that people would somehow feel a sense of connection to each other, whether the connection existed between team members, the patient and the doctor, the nurse and the patient, or the family member and the medical student. To me, all connections were equally important, and would affect patient outcome in the long run.

By now, the nurse had usually joined rounds and the team was confused, overwhelmed, impressed, or all of the above. More importantly, I had made a connection with the patient. We would continue with the physical exam, finish with our plan, and answer questions as promised. Did things always go smoothly? No. Did all patients like me as their doctor? No. I was brutally honest, and had low tolerance for excuses such as "I ran out of my medications," although I would try to find out the root cause for noncompliance. "This is the fifth time you've been admitted in the last year for the same problem, and yet you can afford your cocaine. How is it that you can't afford your medications and can't get a ride to clinic, but you always have the means and the time to continue to find and use cocaine, which is hurting you? All of us here want to help you, but please help us better help you control your disease by taking your medications and stop using cocaine."

Would I raise my voice and get upset? Yes. Did you simply want me to tell you that failure to diagnose pulmonary

MNEMONIC FOR FIRST IMPRESSIONS
AT THE BEDSIDE

Age: Patient appears younger/older than stated age.

Bed Position: Be careful with assumptions related to elevated filling pressure and predicting CHF since the position may be for comfort only.

Consciousness: Is the patient awake, alert, tracking across the room, or laughing at my bad jokes?

Distress: If the patient appears uncomfortable or if he makes you uncomfortable, go ask for help.

Ethnicity: Could the ethnicity affect your differential diagnosis? How about considering sarcoidosis in an African American patient or rheumatic heart disease or pericardial tuberculosis in an immigrant?

Facies: Do you see facial asymmetry, features of Marfan's, Cushing's, xanthelasma, premature arcus, a malar flush, rhinophyma, or perhaps a goiter or prison tattoo with tear drops?

Gender: Is this patient a man, a woman, or transgender, and would that affect your differential diagnosis or your preconceived notions about their presentation? Ask yourself why women who complain of chest pain don't get the same care as men with the identical complaint and presentation.

Habitus: Is the patient tall (Marfan's), thin (weight loss, homeless, drug abuse, malnourished, known to have cancer or metabolic derangements), obese (sleep apnea, insulin resistance accelerating atherosclerosis), or short (perhaps the weight of 150 pounds in a 4-foot 11-inch patient is not healthy)?

embolus and treating the patient as having community-acquired pneumonia was acceptable? When you as the presenter told me the exam was unremarkable, but I found all the physical exam signs of liver cirrhosis, including the fact that the patient was yellower than a lemon, was I supposed to just say it was OK? I couldn't do that. Perhaps I was young and angry. Maybe I was a product of the era I trained in. Was I really a surgeon stuck in internal medicine? *(Please say no, somebody!)*. Did I care too much? Yes. I was full of idealism and desired the same from others. I knew subconsciously that a pat on the back was not too far from a kick in the ass. I believed some learners needed the latter because they'd been pampered with too much of the former.

There was no middle ground. In my early days as an attending, you either loved me or wished I was dead. People either requested to be on my service or begged to not be placed on it. I had so many HOPESFEARSDREAMSTEARS, and yet somehow I was drowning in my own idealism..

My lifeboat had already arrived on December 2, 1996, in the form of my first child, Natasha. And yet I was too consumed in wanting to change the world that I couldn't change myself. Lucky for me, although I tried to crash SS Niraj into many icebergs, my second lifeboat arrived on March 25, 1999, in the form of my second daughter Poonum, when I had worked my way back to LBJ full-time. I remembered a magnet I had seen at Barnes & Noble: "To the world you are one person, but to one person you are the world." How could I be so rough around the edges and still be the "one" for my two beautiful angels? They were my HOPESFEARSDREAMSTEARS. *Krishna, you were right. No Mom and Dad, the patient Krishna, not Krishna Bhagvan.* Something would have to change. I would have to change.

53

Change Is Coming

My heart and my soul Mehta

The baby steps towards change began slowly. I would need, as Rohinton Mistry suggested, "a fine balance" between intention and perception. I didn't want to be perceived as someone that I clearly wasn't. I never made the effort at a conscious level, but the changes were happening at the subconscious level.

When I was young and rebellious, my dad's answer to any question I asked was the same: "Son, you will understand when you have children."

"What the hell does that mean?" I used to ask in a disrespectful tone. He would repeat the mantra like a broken tape recorder or the slokathon from the previous Sunday morning's Chinmaya Mission classes: "Son, you will understand when you have children."

"Enough, old man," I used to say under my breath. I grew tired of this mumbo jumbo classic Indian dad with his "I know what's best for you because I've seen more Diwalis than you" routine. *C'mon Dad, this is life, not a Hindi movie. Give me something objective*, I would think.

"Beta, tu bap banish tyare tu samjish."

"Great, Dad. You said the same thing in Gujarati, and it's still not helpful!"

Like most Indian teenagers growing up in the United States, I eventually gave up, and assumed there was a generational disconnect. I was wrong. My dad was right. My subconscious transformation started with my two children. They had me wrapped around their tiny little fingers, and became my heart and soul from the first glance and fluttering of their eyelashes. In fact years later, when my cell phone rings, it's not their names that appear on the screen but rather "My Heart" and "My Soul," referring to my older and younger daughter, Natasha and Poonam, respectively.

In addition to bringing me an inner sense of calmness, my daughters transformed my office into a sanctuary of nirvana. Before their birth, my office at LBJ was like any other office, I guess, full of diplomas, awards, and other things that mattered to me. As my children grew, I received daily reminders of my dad's cryptic quote in the form of colorful art. Over the years, awards were replaced by drawings from my two little Picassos. Since I'm addicted to ties, my walls were mostly adorned with cut-out ties made in their elementary school for Father's Day. I was quickly running out of wall space. In fact, I started to stick artwork on the ceiling!

I had established a reputation at LBJ as being the toughest attending in medical school and residency. Even with the CARD system, my rounds on the post-call day were long and exhausting. I spent a minimum of eight hours teaching bedside physical exam findings and evidence-based decision-making. As a result, I either pollinated a disciple for life to carry forth the message of healing with equal parts heart and mind—or someone who vowed to never ever spend another day on my service.

Why was my transformation important? By word of

mouth, most learners had preconceived perceptions of me—I assumed most of these were negative—before they started the rotation. A few outliers requested to switch onto my service for the first time, presumably also due to word of mouth by one of my brainwashed disciples.

The office transformation was a reflection of my inner transformation. Why? I gave the orientation speech in my office. It was obvious within the first five minutes that no one was listening to me. All they saw were the drawings, ties, and corny poems and portraits from "My Heart" and "My Soul." I could almost hear the learners' thoughts: *How could such a proud father be a bad guy?* I suspected that they were also thinking about what my previous learners had told me by the end of month: "Dr. Mehta, we had heard all kinds of things about you before this rotation, but you're not what everyone says." I had literally taken baby steps because of my babies. The transformation had begun, and there would be no turning back. Dad, you were right, and now I understand. HOPESFEARSDREAMSTEARS.

54

ID Badges

Pictures are worth a thousand words.

I was changing without realizing it. I was still passionate and could be a mean bastard when a patient's life was at stake. Slowly, however, the glass that was once half empty was transforming itself into one that was always half full.

I was spending my entire academic time at LBJ. Even my clinics had now moved to LBJ Hospital, allowing me to truly maintain continuity between inpatient and outpatient medicine. Unlike traditional primary care models, most of my initial patient encounters took place in the acute care inpatient setting. I would subsequently see the patient in my continuity clinic within two weeks of the patient's hospital discharge. Hospitalized patients were understandably apprehensive when I first met them. As such, I needed to establish trust quickly. "Hello, I'm Dr. Mehta and this is my team. I know you've already seen enough doctors today to last you a lifetime." This was my opening line with every patient encounter. From a singular look in the patient's eyes that matched their nervous smile, I knew that we had made a connection.

I knew enough about diseases but had always believed that the person came first. If I didn't understand Mrs. Johnson as a person who had congestive heart failure and only thought of her in terms of her disease process, I wouldn't be able to help the patient in the long run. As such, my history was initially focused on learning about the patient, not their symptoms. I did this by asking them about life. Was the patient from Houston? If so, where did they go to high school? I knew every local school's mascot name and colors, having spent the last twenty-five years in Houston. If Houston wasn't home, where did the patient grow up, and what was the story behind "I wasn't born in Texas, but I got here as fast as I could?" What did my patient do for a living, and who else was at home? Did the patient have any kids or grandkids? In asking these questions, I was able to establish a connection with even the most guarded of patients. How? No matter how sick the patient was, I always saw a twinkle in their eyes when I asked them about their children or grandchildren. I had carried pictures of my kids in my wallet for years. As a proud father, I would show them pictures of my pride and joy. In return, I would ask to see pictures of their loved ones. If the patient didn't have them, I would remind family members to bring the prized "Kodak memory burn" before rounds the next day.

One day, the light bulb in my head suddenly turned on. What if I moved the pictures from my wallet to my coat? How was that possible? Easy. I would make my kids' pictures my ID badge and carry my required ID badge in my pocket. At Kinko's, I trimmed Natasha's and Poonum's pictures and laminated them. I next clipped the hole in my ID badge and put in the clip tag. Presto, I had an ID badge! I tried my little experiment with the new ID badge, and noticed that my patients' body language in the emergency room mirrored the residents' responses in my office. When I spoke, the first thing they saw as I made eye contact and offered a warm handshake was my kids' pictures. Instant reflection in each patient's eyes from a moment of remembrance, and a lifetime of trust was established in seconds! Over the years, the joke at LBJ was that even the janitor knew what my kids looked like since my new ID badge was visible on my coat twenty-four hours a day, seven days a week.

I changed their pictures every year and still do. Of course, they're now embarrassed, and roll their eyes since they are ages sixteen and fourteen. Although I had separate ID badges for Natasha and Poonum, somehow one would always cover up the other. When they were younger, my kids would take turns claiming that I loved one more than the other, depending upon which picture was more visible. I started to flip the order of visibility every other day to let them know that they were equal in my eyes. As time passed, my students and residents noticed the badges. I would be alerted if I forgot to flip the ID picture badge.

In essence, LBJ had become home, and my patients, students, and residents had become part of my ever growing family. The only constant is change, and I was finally changing for the better. HOPESFEARSDREAMSTEARS.

55

4:30 a.m.

Heaven on earth

My adopted family was growing and work no longer felt like work. I was up at 4:30 a.m. every fourth day, but I was always smiling because I was simply traveling from one home to another. Even my morning routine reflected the change. Preset buttons on my radio were changed from FM to AM. I was listening to infomercials on everything from FOCUS Factor supplements to erectile dysfunction *(stop laughing)*. If no infomercial was on the radio during the early morning drive, no problem. I had an easy solution. I would listen to the hunting and fishing show on 610 AM. The irony? I'm a vegetarian who never considered either hobby, even in my dreams.

Since I lived in Pearland, a suburb of Houston, my drive to LBJ was twenty-seven miles. With all that time in the car, I was becoming an expert on all kinds of vitamins and fishing baits. On the way in for 6:00 a.m. rounds, I would stop by Shipley Do-Nuts on the corner of Highway 288 and Holcombe Boulevard to pick up the morning sugar kick for the team. In doing so, I would periodically encounter some of my former homeless patients that I had long forgotten. They wanted money, but I would buy them a doughnut, a kolache, or a cup of coffee and chat for few minutes before heading off for rounds.

My heart seemed to be constantly growing in size, and that would have made even the Grinch jealous. I guess I would live longer because of it. My slow transformation continued on rounds. I used to drink at least a six-pack of Diet Coke every day, and now I had cut down to four cans per day. And no, I don't want your evidence-based paper on diet drinks, specifically those with high phosphorous content and artificial sweeteners. The team noticed my attempt to cut back, and when I would show up for post-call rounds, they would have a bottle of Diet Coke waiting for me. I guess they must have finally figured out that I didn't get up at 4:30 a.m. just to scream at them, but that somehow I cared about their education. Just like I'd done with the ID badge twinkle, I had connected with the team. In time, the Diet Coke and doughnuts became our bond.

I used to arrive fifteen minutes early and start my little serpentine walk. This would be followed by a moment of silence as I admired the morning light reflecting all of its beautiful colors on the kids' playground on the fourth floor. Having achieved my own transient nirvana, I would open the office door, stare at the priceless art pieces, laugh with the reflexive Pavlovian Bell's palsy smile, and head down to the radiology reading area for rounds. The theme of heaven on earth seemed to repeat itself over and over again as I chuckled, thinking once again about Yogi Berra's famous quote, "It's like déjà vu all over again."

On the last post-call day of the rotation, I would not only bring doughnuts, but also sparkling cider and plastic champagne glasses. I had looked up the sunrise time in advance and adjusted the start time for rounds accordingly. This actually caused a lot of unnecessary heart rate variability for the team because I always followed a schedule. If the routine was broken, it could only mean trouble. As I opened the door to the playground, their fear of the unknown would quickly dissipate. In its place was a dreamlike trance of "I can't believe what I'm seeing." As we drank fake champagne, I was sometimes asked if I could bring the "good stuff" in the future. Everyone would join in the laughter that followed as I started to speak. I would simply thank them for their effort and remind them that I cared. My hope was that they would understand why I worked them so hard. I would leave them with the quote "your journey is your destination" and ask them to appreciate the beauty of the sunrise before the twilight of their career. The sun would slowly rise over the smog-filled horizon, creating a kaleidoscope of colors that was impossible to describe.

Over the years, my champagne always tasted a bit salty, ironically from tears that were so sweet. In such moments, it was as if heaven existed at LBJ, and all my hopes and dreams had come true.

56

Beginning of Writing

Cheaper than Prozac

Serpentine walks, badge pictures of "My Heart" and "My Soul," and sunrise memories became my Prozac. I was changing, hopefully for the better. During this time, I also began to write. It started with random thoughts and observations, at first written on the pink and white sheets of paper from my residency. This quickly turned into writing on my hands or even on cocktail napkins during flights 30,000 feet above ground. Was this a sign of Prozac toxicity? Did I need more Prozac? Was this a midlife crisis? Had I seen the movie *Memento* too many times? *At least I have no tattoos yet*, I used to whisper to myself, *except the scars from old vaccines I had gotten growing up in India*. The last time I enjoyed writing this much was in high school, when I thought I wanted to teach English for a living.

Perhaps it was an outlet, because although I read as many medical journals as I could, what I felt was missing were the stories describing the actual journey of becoming a physician. Maybe I was just reading the wrong journals. Was I just lost and confused? Who was I going to tell about my vague feeling of emptiness? I was too old to tell my parents, even for an Indian kid. My wife? No, thank you. She had already read *Men are from Mars*, *Women are from Venus* and thought I belonged there. My boss, Kojak, the one who had gotten me out of the medical center as fast as he could? Are you kidding? I was already a salmon swimming upstream alone without a paddle. Who needed to hear about my version of *Salmon Fishing in the Yemen* (well actually *Salmon Fishing in Academic Medicine*), especially coming from an Indian. My students and residents? NWJ—No Way, Jose, to use a phrase I borrowed from my undergrad mentor, Dr. Wentland.

If I shared my predicament with the team, I was afraid they'd say, "I knew it. He always tells us Prozac should be in nation's water supply, but he needs it more than anyone else does!" I had one other choice. I could tell my two kids, who would have sat and listened to my sudden intractable DOTM (Diatribe Of The Mouth, as opposed to what you might be thinking the *D* stands for). But I heard Bruce Willis's voice in *Look Who's Talking*: "Oh yeah, he's flipped!" So I kept my mouth shut.

The words, however, kept slowly pouring out of my heart onto a book of previously unwritten pages, and I realized that the final piece of the puzzle was emerging. During my residency, I had always worried that I had forgotten why I became a doctor. Now that I had remembered why, I wanted to write so that I would never forget again.

Writing was like breathing, and now it had become essential for my survival. I wrote about everything from childhood memories to academic disappointments. It started with a quote or a phrase, which would trigger a cascade of pent up subconscious thoughts. It seemed as if these thoughts had been locked away with the hopes that someday someone would find the key. Small bits of wisdom emerged over time, and I started to convert the quotes and phrases into simple poems or short stories. I kept multiple journals, one in my office, one in my car, and one on my bedside table. As these pages were rapidly filled with emotions, a heart of darkness was slowly and finally shedding some light unto the human being I was long before I became a doctor. I hoped that this newly discovered Stealth who had previously been "visibly invisible" would continue to be present long after I finished my academic career. Imagine the opening lines of *Law and Order* as you read the following:

"The doctors of tomorrow are part of a special group of overworked, underpaid angry young men and women who got so busy trying to save the dying that somehow they forgot that they were still living. Here are their stories."

Perhaps you can even tap on something next to you for effect, similar to the show's opening credits. I started sharing stories and poems with my students, residents, and nurses, hoping that perhaps others needed Prozac as much as I did. Assuming that you live in a part of our country that also has low levels of Prozac in the water supply, I have shared some of these stories and poems with you here.

The Cupcake Man

Having trained at a local county hospital in Houston, Texas, I was always taught first the value of limited resources. At the time, it was difficult to understand that I was training in the world's largest medical center, yet most of my patients would never be afforded the luxury of the technological advances that I was exposed to during lectures and noon conferences. I was able to diagnose many diseases as if they had popped out of *Harrison's Principles of Internal Medicine* straight onto my ward service. Unfortunately, I could diagnose only so much before the paper chart during my training resembled Tolstoy's *War and Peace.*

Over time, I began to wonder about the point of making a diagnosis if I couldn't relieve the patient's suffering by actually treating that disease. There was, of course, one exception to that rule at The County. The key was looking at more than a patient's name on the identification stamp of every chart.

The first thing I noticed as an intern looking at Tolstoy's recurrent masterpiece was what my upper-level resident had taught me: "Make sure you look to see if they have a second smaller number on the identification stamp, because if they do, then they have secondary insurance, and we can actually help them!" I never took care of those with private insurance, because those patients would not be admitted to a county hospital, for obvious reasons. However, I would encounter some patients with Medicare Parts A and/or B. The local county access card was known as a gold card, but if I saw the secondary number, I would label my patient as the one having the platinum card.

As time passed, I noticed that the number of patients with a gold card far exceeded those with the platinum card. What could I do to help the masses that would never be able to receive the therapeutic expertise located down the street at MD Anderson Cancer Center or the Texas Heart Institute? I was reminded of what an older attending who still wore bowties had once told me, though at the time, it didn't seem important. "Heal with your heart and your mind and you will heal your patients, not just their disease." Easy for someone to say who didn't have the twenty-four hours on and twenty-four hours off shift in the emergency room, or have to admit twenty patients in a twenty-four hour span.

As the third year of residency started, I continued to look for secondary insurance on the identification stamp of every patient. Cynicism was in full bloom, and frankly I wasn't a nice person. Sadly, I fit in with the rest of my colleagues, and the only ones suffering from our combined arrogance were the patients.

One day I saw something new in those identification stamps: Instead of how many more years until the patient's sixty-fifth birthday, which would qualify them for Medicare, I noticed the actual date of birth. My patient was having his birthday in the hospital today! I even noticed his name. His name was John.

The quote from Dr. Bowtie came flooding back. I ran to the cafeteria and bought a small cupcake. I returned to John's bedside and offered it to him. He asked me if I would sing him a song. I sang "Happy Birthday" and saw his eyes fill with tears. He wasn't alone, for the nurse and I also noticed that the twin lakes on our faces were also flooded with an overwhelming sense of joy. It was as if we had somehow found a way to help the gold card patient feel as if he were a platinum member of society. That day, I labeled John "The Cupcake Man."

Over time, I have modified the birthday ceremony. The cupcake now includes candles, and may come in different flavors depending on the patient's preference. We also sing

"Happy Birthday" in the patient's native language. We're far from successful, and have even been known to butcher it. However, it always brings a smile.

I have now become Dr. Bowtie, although I don't wear a bowtie. I'm rapidly advancing in my age in this era of sophisticated technology with electronic medical records and a multitude of diagnostic and therapeutic applications available even at The County. I know because I still work at the same hospital district I trained in. When I ask my learners the first thing they notice when they look at a medical chart, not a single student or resident has ever replied "the patient's birth date"—that is, until recently. The question was asked by me during bedside rounds and the answer came from the patient.

"You should pay attention to him and pay attention to my birth date," said the patient. I was astonished not only at what the patient just stated but at what my eyes noticed next.

It was The Cupcake Man, John. "Hi Doc, it's been a while. Birthday is still off a few months, but who knows maybe I'll be back for my cupcake." He went on to tell the inpatient team our story from over fifteen years ago, and not a dry eye was left in the audience.

We often wonder during our training why we do what we do, second-guessing our reasons for becoming a doctor. We often struggle as educators in our efforts to convince residents that their journey is their destination. Somewhere along the way, we will understand, hopefully, that the power of helping and healing comes in many different forms. For me that day, it came in the form of The Cupcake Man.

WWJD

In an era of eighty-hour work weeks for residents combined with the constant expectation that the attending physician be a triple threat—researcher, clinician, and teacher—it is not uncommon to have the medical student as the sole team member providing continuity of care on an inpatient teaching service. The adaptive team structure has led to on-the-fly teaching moments usually dictated by the attending and the upper-level resident. Rarely had a student been the teacher, until the day I met Jason.

Jason was like most of his classmates who had just started their clinical rotations. He was quiet, honest, hardworking, and slowly trying to grasp clinical medicine. This was no easy feat, especially when internal medicine was his first rotation at a busy county hospital. About ten days into the rotation, I was told by Jason that our patient, Tom, who had severe peripheral vascular disease and progressive multiple non-healing bilateral ulcers of the feet, was reluctant to have surgical intervention to restore circulation. I saw an opportunity for an on-the-fly teaching moment and decided to take the team to Tom's room.

For the next fifteen minutes, I discussed in detail the hospital course to date, the previous recurrent admissions for the same problem, the need for surgical intervention, and the depth-perception picture of what may happen in the future. I was hopeful that such a discussion by a triple threat would perhaps help alleviate any doubts or concerns that Tom may have had. I was wrong.

I asked Tom if he had any questions, concerns, comments, or suggestions. He told me that he didn't. When I asked him if this meant that he was ready for the surgical procedure, he paused and looked at Jason. "Well now, that depends on what my doctor here tells me to do. Tell 'em, Doc. I trust you more than any of these guys 'cause you're the only one who spends time with me every day."

I thought Jason was going to collapse from heart rate variability, as was the rest of the team. I simply smiled and reflected on how I had been a part of a spontaneous teaching moment. My teacher was my medical student, Jason.

Tom did have the procedure the next morning, and it was because of his doctor, Jason. That day, I learned that teaching moments are unpredictable, but that Jason was a better teacher than I, for he was responding to the needs of his patient. Meanwhile, I was too busy treating peripheral vascular disease with ulcers. On the last day of the rotation, I gave Jason a wrist band that read WWJD. He asked me what this had to with religion. I showed him my identical wrist band and reminded him that the initials stood for What Would Jason Do.

Gifted students become teachers, but more importantly, teachers are reminded at times that they must be lifelong students. I will be a lifelong student of Jason, and ten years into a career as a full-time medical educator, I still ask myself every day *WWJD?*

If

If you could see through my eyes,
You would not see diabetic retinopathy,
But a grandfather who could not see a baseball game with his grandson.

If you could hear what I hear,
You would not hear aortic stenosis,
But a woman who could no longer enjoy working in her garden.

If you could touch what I touch,
You would not touch an infected wound,
But a woman with an impending amputation
Losing hope of evening walks with her husband.

If you could smell what I smell,
You would not smell the stench of chronic diarrhea,
But be overwhelmed with a sense of dignity lost
And embarrassment felt for a grown man in a diaper.

You think you see, and yet you are blind.
You think you hear,
But so does the patient your words so unkind.

Do you see what you have become?
A cynical, self-absorbed arrogant pawn.

Hippocrates cried a tear today.
For you left another M & M Conference happy and gay.

Sit with your patient, ask him why.
And you might learn something
From a sage reflecting on time gone by.

Give him a hug and make him smile,
And you will realize your day was worthwhile.

So rise to the challenge
And from this moment your indifference must cease.
Before it's too late my young friend,
And your tombstone also says rest in peace.

My Students

What would you rather be, to my students I ask,
Hoping to discover the soul beneath the mask.

For it is their stories I wish to know,
To remove the rust and restore their inner glow.

Are they from small towns, eyes full of hope?
If so, remind them ambition is a slippery slope.

Do they really want to be here and if so why,
For living an unfulfilled life is the easiest way to die.

Are they focused yet well-rounded?
For patient's perception of an MD's arrogance is rarely unfounded.

Are they wound too tight like ticking clocks?
If so, a joke will remind them laughter (is the key that) opens all
locks.

Do they appear aloof and smug?
Let them melt in the arms of a patient with a hug.

Give them freedom to learn from a mistake,
But remind them sternly that a life was at stake.

Lessons, lessons so many lessons to be learned,
For my students are my role models, my Honors to be earned.

The Bench

They call it winds of change;
But how can that be if it all looks the same.

I sat on this weathered wooden bench
in need of a new stain in 1989.
Now I sit again in 2004.

Back then, an idealistic medical student;
Today an idealistic attending.

The building looks the same, so do the trees;
Even the dews of water falling from the leaves.

Yes, it all looks the same.
The only difference;
I used to sit on this wooden bench
more often instead of chasing life's fleeting fortune and fame.

Today, I see the reflection only because I reflect;
On the years I spent passing the bench in neglect.

57

Funerals

Mr. BP's sunrise and sunset

I was still imperfect, but unlike before, was adapting to my limitations. Understanding my own shortcomings had made me a better academic physician and teacher. For so long, I had lacked the courage to recognize and reconcile my imperfections as well as those of my environment. But everything was changing.

I was learning that sadly, all the efforts in the world could not always save a patient's life. I had followed some of my patients in the clinic since I was a resident, and when one of these patients died, it was as if a piece of me died with them. I tried to make sense of what went wrong and if I could've done anything differently to change the outcome. To provide my aching heart with closure—as NNN's brutally honest quote kept creeping back into my mind ("Niraj, you never learn from your mistakes because you bury them")—I started to attend my patients' funerals. I was skeptical of my own decision, though. Why was I doing this? *Was I crazy?*

Most doctors don't go to their patients' funerals. What would I do if a family member told me that their loved one died because of me? Was I really going to bury a mistake?

Was this part of the Kübler-Ross sequence? What would people think of me as the only Indian person in a predominantly African American crowd? Would I have a heart of stone or would the twin lakes on my face overflow with embarrassing leaky faucets that I could not control nor turn off?

Although my emotions were a mixed bag of confusion, I couldn't help myself from going. I tried to be discreet, hoping that no one would recognize me. I always sat in the corner of the last row, trying to blend into a background of invisibility, reading "Sunrise to Sunset," as the program was often entitled, about the life and death of my patient.

The first funeral I attended was for a patient who had died of a massive heart attack. I remember the first time I had met him in clinic. As usual, he was the last patient of the day. He had no medical records and had lost his insurance—he could thus not afford to pay for his medications—and now would be seen at LBJ. Murphy may be an Irish name, but his law seemed to be housed at the LBJ clinic and always included a patient like this one. Did I mention this patient's blood pressure had been 235/122, and he was just sitting there patiently waiting to be seen? I had yelled at nurses and residents to remind them not to treat any number in the clinic—most importantly, a blood pressure elevation—without an objective evaluation by a doctor. This was especially relevant to the term hypertensive urgency since the urgency seemed to involve controlling the nurse and doctor's heart rate as opposed to the patient's blood pressure. However, this particular patient's unusually high number was elevating even my subconscious blood pressure. As such, the resident and I decided to see the patient immediately.

Although the patient was stable and asymptomatic, it was obvious from my physical exam that he had chronic end organ damage from his longstanding uncontrolled and presumed primary hypertension. He had a tapping apex beat the size of a quarter grossly displaced downward and out towards the anterior axillary line. All of his heart valves seemed to be leaking, and his entire precordium seemed to be one loud murmur that I couldn't distinguish beyond "systolic" without an increase with Valsalva maneuver (thus eliminating the likelihood of hypertrophic obstructive cardiomyopathy or mitral valve prolapse). He had two extra heart sounds, one in systole and one in diastole.

I tried to change his bed position and made an effort to listen for murmurs with the patient in the left lateral decubitus position and then leaning forward in end-expiration. The upper-level resident was clearly enjoying himself because I took pride in my exam and he could tell I was confused as to what the hell I was listening to. The patient's pulses were noted to be symmetric and without delay but hyperdynamic, as would be expected given the increased afterload in the form of hypertension. Everywhere I listened, though, I could hear a murmur, but that was impossible! Why? Sadly, as I had used the term before during rounds, this man was a "bruit machine" head to toe, starting from his carotids, moving down to his abdomen, and finally his femoral arteries! The exam concluded with an S3, S4, a right ventricular heave, a left atrial lift, a loud P2, elevated jugular venous pressure, a winking ear lobe sign, a pulsatile liver, and gross bilateral pitting edema with prolonged pit recovery time.

This patient might as well have been wearing a t-shirt that stated the obvious, "I have congestive heart failure." Although I had done my best to reassure the patient during my introduction ("Hello, Mr. BP. I'm Dr. Mehta and this is Dr. Patel. I'm sure you have seen enough doctors to last you a lifetime, but I'm going to spend a few minutes here to talk to you and examine you. It may take some time, and part of my job is to teach so please don't be alarmed if I spend extra time for example listening to your heart. Do not assume this means something is wrong. If I make you uncomfortable at any time, please stop me,

otherwise again I will try to explain to you when I finish what the problem is and how I can try to help you"), he must have guessed from my puzzled face, the detailed exam, and other nonverbal clues that something was wrong. I guess he would've made a great doctor.

I continued as usual to be a bad poker player, unable to hide my "tells." Mr. BP noticed the expression on my face but had been quiet as I finished the exam. I was about to start talking when he politely interjected, "First of all doctor, thank you for seeing me today and I think we're going to get along fine because you value the same thing I do in all interactions, which is trust and relationship. You see, I noticed the pictures, I assume of your kids, on your coat pocket when you walked in, and although I'm the last patient on a late Friday afternoon, you're not in a hurry to get me out of here. So, again thank you for helping me. And now tell me why you've done such a complete exam and have a concerning, puzzled look on your face."

I was, of course, lost for words—albeit temporarily— as Patel kept smiling like the lead actor Salman Khan in an Indian movie. Was I the patient and was this patient my psychiatrist? I quickly gathered my composure and explained to him that my team was on call and that we would admit him to the hospital to improve his blood pressure. We would also investigate the potential causes as well as the likelihood of chronic damage, due to his hypertension, to different parts of his body, including the concerning findings on my exam suggesting damage to his heart. I used the kid glove approach so as not to alarm Mr. BP, as Emily Dickinson started whispering in my head:

Hope is the thing with feathers
That perches in the soul,
And sings the tune--without the words,
And never stops at all,

And sweetest in the gale is heard;
And sore must be the storm
That could abash the little bird
That kept so many warm.

I've heard it in the chillest land,
And on the strangest sea;
Yet, never, in extremity,
It asked a crumb of me

I admitted the patient to the hospital, and started the simultaneous process of investigating the cause of the hypertension and likely resultant congestive heart failure and accelerated systemic arteriosclerosis. An extensive evaluation to look for a secondary cause of his chronic hypertension was unremarkable. Unfortunately, although bruits by themselves are of no clinical consequence in an asymptomatic patient, their presence in Mr. BP represented the probability of accelerated arteriosclerosis. Imaging studies confirmed our suspicions. He had blockage of bilateral carotid arteries, bilateral femoral arteries, distal unilateral renal artery stenosis without asymmetric dilation of kidneys, and diffuse atherosclerosis of his abdominal and thoracic aorta with gross calcification and non-critical aneurysmal dilation. His echo confirmed severe bilateral congestive heart failure with secondary leakage of all four heart valves. He had diffuse coronary artery disease with poor target vessels, and he was thus deemed "medical management."

All internists know but refuse to admit—it has taken me almost twenty years to admit it—that surgeons have the most common sense in the world when it comes to doctors and are not afraid of anything. As such, when a surgeon writes on the chart "medical management," this is a code phrase for either "why the hell did you call this stupid consult?" or "your patient is screwed, sorry." In this case, the answer obviously reflected the latter and not the former.

To prevent further progression of his disease, I continued to be aggressive with Mr. BP's care in terms of primary prevention. I kept a close eye on him and his data points during multiple subsequent clinic visits. He knew his disease well, and fondly labeled himself "a learning bruit machine" when I would periodically send in new residents or medical students to examine him during clinic visits. He was human. Although he tried his best, he would inevitably be admitted to my inpatient service for what I called "pizza failure" due to dietary indiscretions, especially during the holiday season. He always apologized and, because I had slowly come to grips with my own imperfections over time, I was more forgiving than I had been during my residency years. In fact, I would be upset with residents for using the term "noncompliant" with his diet or "frequent flyer" since he was admitted often to the hospital service. I urged them to understand the reason for Mr. BP's "noncompliance" and the natural progression of his disease, which was driven more by nature than by nurture.

Why have I spent so much time talking about Mr. BP in detail? Unfortunately, it is to highlight how little I knew about Mr. BP, in spite of all the details I thought I knew about him. I knew his history. I knew his exam. I knew all of his laboratory data. I knew all his imaging studies. I knew all of his consultative opinions. I even knew when I had last seen him in clinic or in the hospital down to the specific date. Yet I didn't know him.

At his funeral, I discovered that while I knew

everything I needed to know about hypertension and atherosclerosis, I didn't know Mr. BP. I knew the disease, but not the patient. His eulogy started with remembrance of a man who taught statistics at University of Houston. *He did?* I thought. *Maybe that's why he was so observant and analytical about his disease progression.* I think he was well aware of his long-term prognosis.

The speaker continued. Mr. BP was an All-American swimmer at the University of Texas. *He was?!* Someone sitting next to me gave me an admonishing look. Apparently, my thoughts of disbelief had unknowingly been vocalized, and once again betrayed my confidence. I didn't know Mr. BP at all. I was embarrassed and ashamed.

Now it was his sister's turn to talk. "Most of you know that we come from a humble background and were born dirt poor. However, what you may not have known is that I wouldn't have gotten to go to my prom if it wasn't for my brother."

Yeah, I know, I was thinking, *he was your date. How kind?*

She must have been a mind reader because she continued. "And, no, he wasn't my prom date."

"Damn it," I blurted out.

"Young man, you are in the house of God!" said my neighbor again.

I was clenching my teeth, hoping that this would keep me from opening my mouth.

"No, the reason I couldn't go to prom was that I couldn't afford a prom dress. But my brother Mr. BP saw me crying, and he actually sewed a dress for me using discarded material from a local seamstress."

I was still clenching my teeth, but my mind was screaming, *What the hell? I'm a completely useless physician,* as by now the faucets that I was afraid of were starting to open up on my face. I was so distraught that I could not remember the rest of the eulogy. Afterwards, as I tried to sneak out incognito, I was stopped by Mr. BP's sister.

"Hello, you must be Dr. Mehta?"

Huh? No, I'm the idiot who took care of your brother for over five years but didn't know anything about him. My teeth were still clenched, so fortunately that thought didn't come out. "Yes, I am," I responded.

"I know we never met, but my family and I just want to thank you so much for taking such great care of him. He always talked about you, especially during the holiday season dinners with my family, because he told us that he would probably be at LBJ for some extra fluid pills over the next three days and that the only doctor who would understand why without judging him was you."

Damn it, faucets! Tears were flowing down my face. "He also told us you are very hard on your residents, but it's because you care and want to help but just don't know how." I was standing there like a statue seeing my previous patient Krishna reincarnated in front of me. I think she saw the tears and my inability to force words out. She gave me a hug and told me, "We love you."

With a heart that was now a wet sponge, I slowly walked out of the church, thanking the family that had joined the sister in a parade of hugs. I had come to LBJ hoping to change one life at a time through patient care and education. Instead, LBJ and all that it represented had slowly changed the one person who was not capable of changing himself: me. HOPESFEARSDREAMS and lots and lots of TEARS.

58

Mr. Luby's

Professor of humanity and humility

It's hard to imagine what working at a county hospital was like back in the day unless you were there. For most of us who are not doctors, our image of a county hospital is the classic lead story of the evening news. At least that's the way it was in Houston. "Another gunshot wound" was the 10:00 p.m. lead news story, and "the patient was taken to a local county hospital in critical condition." Another version was the "high speed police chase involving a drug dealer that ended in a tragic accident with the suspect now in critical condition at a local county hospital."

From the outside, the world compartmentalized the county hospital as a place for taking care of lazy, uninsured patients or a place for homeless substance abusers and prisoners. The doctors were mostly in training or came from other countries as foreign medical graduates. Both groups would clearly prefer to be somewhere else if they had been given a choice. The general public had a similar opinion. Do you ever want to be admitted to a county hospital? In fact, many taxpayers still feel as if their dollars are taking care of those who don't want to help themselves. Although there are rotten apples who abuse every system and The County clearly has its share, I was constantly inspired by the stories I witnessed firsthand at LBJ, especially as an attending perhaps headed towards neurotransmitter changes heralding a "midlife crisis."

One such story came in the form of a patient I called Luby's because he had a buffet platter of diseases including COPD, hepatitis C, diabetes mellitus, hypertension, hyperlipidemia, hypothyroidism status post radioactive ablation for Graves' disease, monoclonal gammopathy of unknown significance, chronic renal insufficiency, benign prostatic hypertrophy, diastolic and congestive heart failure. Did I mention that he also had chronic severe asymmetric venous stasis due to his job driving trucks for over forty years, ten hours a day for seven days a week in the prime of his life? In fact, I used to laugh because the new interns would present him to me during clinic rounds and tell me that his chief complaint was "I don't have a blood clot in my leg so don't order another ultrasound!"

We connected over the years and somehow I was able to convince him to give up tobacco—no small task, especially at LBJ. He always traveled and would sometimes be on the road for three months at a time. I had learned my lesson from Mr. BP, so I knew Luby's story well. He lived in the country on a ranch. We talked about how he would take me on his truck for travel up north at no cost to me since his lungs seemed to act up in cold weather. I would be his traveling doctor. We joked about how I would visit him on his ranch, where he barbecued, once he retired. The joke was that I would ask him to make tofu burgers and skewers. Of course, he had no idea I was vegetarian or what the heck tofu was until I told him.

He talked about how he missed fishing with his brother, who had passed away. I told him about how I had gone fishing once in the seventh grade and had let go of the only goldfish I caught. We laughed, and I promised him that I would be his doctor as long as he would allow me to do so. Laughingly, he reminded me that I was going to be a doctor much longer than he was going to be my patient.

I was slowly getting older, and by extension so were my patients like Luby's, whose plethora of chronic diseases progressed regardless of compliance on the part of the patient, or the efforts of his doctor, and everyone else involved. One day, Luby's had a massive heart attack and was taken to a prestigious medical center hospital. He had life-saving bypass heart surgery and proudly returned to the clinic to show me his scar three months later. I assumed he had been traveling and that was the reason for his missed clinic appointments. I wanted to scream at the thought of not having done the best I could for him, but by now I knew the history of unstable plaques and their pathophysiology. As such, I told him I was glad that he was alive, but he should have called me.

We didn't have a dedicated nurse line at the time at LBJ, but I encouraged all clinic patients to contact me or the lead resident anytime through the page operator. He smiled when I reminded him of this, nodded in agreement, and asked me for a favor I'll never forget. "Dr. Mehta, you know I don't have insurance and the heart hospital saved my life. They think I'm disabled, but I want you to un-disable me so I can work another couple of years and pay them back for saving my life."

I was so tired by now of others taking away my right to DOTM that nothing seemed to surprise me. And yet here I was once again speechless.

"You ok, Dr. Mehta? You look a little browner than usual and you might turn black like me if you keep this up." He laughed in his raspy, hoarse voice.

I looked at him and again Dr. Wentland came to mind,

but I was thinking NWJ (No Way, Jose). He responded, "I know what you're going to say."

Great, another mind reader, I said to myself. *How many of you are out there?*

"I promise I'll cut back on work, but you gotta let me go back."

I refused. I knew he was too sick to work.

Another three months passed and after repeated answers of "no" from me, I broke down and allowed him to fulfill his wishes. *Why the hell is a story like this never on the evening news?* I asked myself, angry once again about people's preconceived notions of the "lazy" patients at The County.

Luby's continued to work and paid back nearly all of his financial debt to the hospital before he passed away to the big ranch in the sky. I sometimes still hear his voice and see his smiling face while flipping tofu burgers when I look up towards the clouds. His heart was as large as a Luby's buffet platter, and his memory serves as a daily reminder of how my patients at The County were professors of humanity and humility for all of us.

59

My Savior

N of 1 has power.

Sometimes a person's professional journey is forever altered by one person more so than any other. For me, it came in the form of My Savior, a patient with severe chronic congestive heart failure due to cocaine abuse. I had always been extremely critical of patients choosing to live an unhealthy lifestyle, especially one related to drug abuse, until I met My Savior. She was a frequent flyer who bounced from clinic to clinic and from one service to another with the same diagnosis and labels, including "noncompliance."

She was now admitted to my inpatient team. The residents knew the fastest way to send a patient home was to inform me that the urine drug screen was positive for cocaine. At the time, I believed that unless a patient was acutely dying, I would not be able to change likely chronic substance abuse that had led to multiple medical problems. I was wrong. As I walked into the room to demonstrate to the team the physical exam findings of congestive heart failure on My Savior, all I could see instead were numerous handmade drawings of "I love you" and "get well soon" that surrounded her bed. The pictures were made by her daughter. We had an instant connection. She saw the pictures of my daughters on the ID badge, and her eyes lit up. We spent the next fifteen minutes talking about our families. This is when I learned that she came from a broken home, was a single mom, and had made horrible choices early in her life, including but not limited to using cocaine.

She told me horrific details about her childhood as my heart bled tears on the inside, hoping my eyes would not give away my secret. I was wrong again, and asked a patient for the first time in all my years, "May I give you a hug?" She told me that other than her daughter, no one else had ever given her a hug. Overwhelmed with emotions, we hugged for what seemed to be forever. As I turned to leave, she wouldn't let go. She told me that she would do whatever it took, but "Please Doctor, help me." She said that although she had stopped using cocaine for years that no one believed her. "Please help me. I want to live for my little girl. I will do whatever you ask of me."

I told her that I wasn't sure if I could do anything different, but would be happy to see her in clinic. So I began seeing My Savior in clinic. I had reminded her that she could not miss any of her appointments and that I would randomly perform urine drug screens to evaluate for substance abuse. I wanted to make sure our trust would not be broken. I also told her that she would need to take all her medications, bring them to the clinic, and record daily weights at home so that we could adjust her medications accordingly. She became my model patient and in time I came up with a plan to help her. I worked with social workers—God's daily reminder of humility on this earth—at LBJ to completely disable My Savior and began the paperwork to qualify her for Medicaid. This process took about six months. Once Medicaid was obtained, I was able to place My Savior on the cardiac transplant list at a hospital in the medical center since she now technically had "insurance" in the form of Medicaid. She continued to see me at the LBJ Internal Medicine Clinic and always introduced me as "this is my savior."

Because of her, over the years I disabled multiple patients to help them get Medicaid. I would then turn over their care to subspecialists in the medical center, since insured patients always had a larger arsenal of treatment options that were not always available to those at The County. Sadly, My Savior died waiting for a heart transplant. The irony of her calling me her savior was never lost on me, for in reality, she was *my* savior. Perhaps evidence-based medicine requires a large patient population and formal studies with enough "power" to suggest a clinically relevant difference in outcome with intervention. My Savior reminded me that although that may be true for diseases, it is not true for patients. All you need is an *N* of 1. Every day at The County, my *N* was growing, and so were my HOPESFEARSDREAMSTEARS.

60

Awards

Priceless promotions

I had been at LBJ for so long now that it had become a part of me. I was content to do the things that were important to me, and my performance in these areas was the yardstick I used to measure my success. I was happy to build a house one brick at a time—or in this case, one human relationship at a time. NNN was still around and teased me that the house I was working on would take "a damn long time to build and probably never be finished." I used to respond with, "But it will be beautiful when it's finished because it will be built on the most important foundation of human relationships, whether it's doctor-patient or student-teacher—or even mentor-protégé like you and I."

"You know Niraj, they must be right, because you're even starting to sound like me although you're not as good looking as me. And by the way, enlighten me with your eastern philosophy mumbo jumbo—what is that most important thing?"

"Trust," I would reply. He smiled and reminded me that he would continue to selfishly take credit for my so-called success. He pointed to his desk where the herd of elephants sat, a gift I had given him several years earlier. I was no longer a part of the herd, and had finally broken away. We laughed, and my heart skipped a beat as I closed his office door, grinning from huge elephant ear to huge elephant ear, having learned over the years "many hear, few listen."

My success never did come in the traditional academic sense. I was never going to be the triple threat academician. I was never going to be lecturing around the world. One brick at a time, remember? So, what was my measuring stick? It was my office and how it was still changing. I already mentioned the steady stream of award-winning masterpieces of art from my two daughters. Over time, the office filled with gifts from those bricks that I had somehow touched over the years. I had lots of ID badges as gifts. Confused? Over the years, the teams I led at LBJ began to take their own picture as a group. The picture would be turned into an ID badge, and handed to me at the end of the rotation with the following quote: "We will never forget you and we hope you will never forget us. Thank you." *Success? Check.*

Since my undergrad days, I had used mnemonics as part of my goofy way of remembering facts. Now that I was a teacher, I had a mnemonic for almost everything, usually running from A to Z. As such, another group of residents actually gave me a group of building blocks with letters as a thank you. *Honors earned? Check.*

Since I was getting older, my notes were sometimes cryptic (thanks, Harvard) and I noticed puzzled looks on rounds the next day. For example, a note might say, "Data collection continues as we try to determine if this patient is a fan of William Shakespeare." When I was politely asked what this strange note meant, I dryly replied, "TB or not TB," given the pulmonary infiltrates that were seen in the upper lobes on the admission chest x-ray. The team rolled their eyes as I chuckled at their response.

One day a student reminded me that the TV show *House* recently had an episode entitled "TB or not TB."

"What? Are you serious? That is my phrase," I said. "I coined it as an intern. Go look at the charts in the warehouse from 1994," I joked.

The resident quipped, "You know, Dr. Mehta, it shouldn't surprise you. You are pretty much like House."

Two security guards were stationed close to us, watching patients in the next room who happened to be from jail. Overhearing our conversation, they now joined in. "That's it, Doc. I knew it. We've known you for years, but couldn't figure out who you remind us of. Your resident is right. You are House."

Like those who had previously called me a "surgeon personality," I wasn't sure if I was being complimented or insulted, especially when the entire team broke into laughter. At the end of that month, I was given my own personal walking cane just like House. Inscribed on the cane were the words "TB or not TB that is the question." To Dr. Mehta, our own House." *Promotion earned? Check.*

I was teaching a significant number of international graduates. We loved reading and chatting over coffee and sweets. Over time, I was given coffee beans from all over the world, gifts from residents who traveled back home for the summer or short vacation breaks. My black java would be accompanied by sweets like Turkish Delights or chikkies, a form of peanut brittle from India with saffron and different nuts. The books? Even the bookshelf was full, and I had to remove the medical textbooks to make room for everything from *Love in the Time of Cholera* to *Midnight Children* to *Osler*. Magnets, paintings, philosophical sayings, and sand sculptures filled my office. *Heaven on earth? Check.*

What about the patients? I took care of restaurant

owners who brought food to the clinic, and we sometimes cheated for a moment on our diabetic diet as we shared forbidden food. We laughed, imagining that God made us diabetics since we were "sweeter than the rest of the world." My patients at LBJ were always financially strapped, but they wanted to give me something in return for my effort. My favorite patient gift? One year for Christmas, I received a gift basket. Inside were twenty empty pill bottles. Homemade labels were affixed to the bottles with written directions. On each bottle's label, the patient had described the actions of a good doctor:

"Take my hand and look into my eyes when you are talking to me."

"Close the curtain to give me privacy when you are examining me in the emergency room."

"Don't be afraid to tell me what you think, I'm human just like you."

"Words may hurt, but your body language can hurt me more."

"Raise the level of the bed so you are not looking down on me."

"Careful what you say outside the door. You may be right, but I have feelings too."

The irony? She was listening because these were quotes that I had used with students and residents on rounds multiple times, reminding them to be a human first and a doctor second. Like most other attendings, I had craved some type of recognition for my efforts, especially in the form of major awards from my department or medical school. Upon visiting my office at LBJ, my dad once stated, "Take a look around. All you need is right here."

Ah, the wisdom of age and the energy of youth. Some honors, like the board exams in internal medicine every ten years, feed your ego and reinforce your belief that you belong. Other forms of honors are like chicken soup *(fine, Mom and Dad, like vegetarian black bean soup)* that nourishes the soul daily. The simple gestures in the form of personalized gifts became, over time, all the awards I ever needed to nourish my belly and my soul. HOPESFEARSDREAMSTEARS.

61

Becoming a Parent

"You remind us of Mom and Dad."

Like many other supposedly complimentary exchanges ("Dr. Mehta, you're like a surgeon"), another common theme was emerging the longer I worked at The County. Students and residents alike would often say, "You remind us of our mom and dad."

Wait a minute, I was thinking. *How do you know that I use hair gel so that all my white hairs will stick together in their stealth mode?* I was already aware of my enlarging forehead, the effects of a receding hairline, which my kids affectionately termed the big head-little hair effect. I suspected Kojak was secretly happy about this. But now students too had taken notice? Was the rapidly enlarging bald spot at the back of my head—which looked like the worn baseline at Wimbledon center court after two weeks of matches—showing its, um, age?

I think the students and residents were probably thinking all of the above but were too polite to tell me directly. Me? I was always direct. So, I asked them. "What exactly do you mean by Mom and Dad?"

"Well, you raise your voice when you're upset, but like you tell us during orientation, it's because you care. Just like our Mom and Dad, you feel disappointed when you believe we could've done better. You have a distraught look on your face as if you feel bad for perhaps hurting our feelings. In the end, however, you know that tough love will eventually work."

How many mind readers are out there? I was thinking to myself. This is why I never understood the players' moves on the World Series of Poker on ESPN. I don't have a good poker face.

"You're always trying to lighten the mood even if at times it is at your own expense," they explained.

I'm a big fan of music and had once tried to connect with students by mentioning the rock band Night Ranger from my high school days. One student responded, "I think I know them. I was in kindergarten when my older brother used to listen to them!"

I didn't know if I wanted to slap him, fail him, or both, but instead I laughed and said, "I meant Blue Oyster Cult, but that would have been on my 8-track recorder before you were born. I guess I'm getting old."

The team would laugh at me, with me, above me, below me, beside me, and behind me, but most importantly, they were laughing. Just when I thought that learners were done with their parental comparisons, others in the group joined in.

"Yeah, you like to tell stories and you always use all this philosophy on rounds with quotes by Shakespeare, Hemingway, Dickinson, and T.S. Eliot. You send us articles on things relevant to patient care, but also about things that make us laugh like "Queer People Enjoying Anatomy" from *The Lancet*, or make us cry like David Millar from *Annals of*

Internal Medicine, or inspire like that funny word I can't pronounce."

"Eraritjaritjaka," I responded.

"Yeah, that's it, whatever you said."

I guess it made sense. I now had two kids and had been an attending for over ten years. What I used to say in jest when I started had actually come true: Medicine is my hobby, but teaching is my passion. Like every other parent, I had in a sense become a dad in more ways than one—instructing, loving, scolding, nurturing, and inspiring.

HOPESFEARSDREAMSTEARS and
ERARITJARITJAKA, indeed.

62

High Expectations

Perceptions over Intentions

My days of double majoring in philosophy and fatherhood, with a minor in being an MD, continued at LBJ. I would be remiss if I failed to mention that the journey was paved with many obstacles. I wasn't always right, but I always demanded evidence for everyone's actions. If a test was ordered, I wanted to know the indications, the pretest probability, and the likelihood that it would change a patient's outcome. Was the test cost-effective? Cost analysis was particularly important to me as a teacher and clinician at LBJ where our resources were limited.

Over the years, the residents had acquired the habit of simply ordering a cornucopia of tests without rhyme or reason. I had been just as guilty of these shortcuts until Harvard and NNN had sparked my own transformation. Since many of these lab tests were ordered without any consideration of pretest probability, no one, including the attending, knew how to interpret the results. The simple solution to such a dilemma? We would just call the consultative services, who as you might expect, ordered additional tests. A classic example of this monkey see monkey do approach involved the ordering of a hepatitis panel for a patient with liver cirrhosis. The panel would tell us if the patient had previous exposure to hepatitis A, B, or C. When I asked the residents how many hepatitis A patients they had seen who developed cirrhosis, the answer was usually, "I haven't seen any." When I asked why, the answer was usually, after some hesitancy, "Because I guess patients with hepatitis A have acute complications but don't develop cirrhosis."

"Then why do you keep ordering a hepatitis panel?" I'd continue.

"Because that's what we've always been taught."

"By whom?"

The answer was always "they." Now I have been looking for "they" for almost twenty years, and still haven't found they, er, them. Sadly, it is because "they" is "us," the medical educators. How will our learners agree on anything when we as teachers don't agree on anything? The idea isn't to take away the art of medicine or individuality. I'm not endorsing the practice of cookie-cutter medicine, but shouldn't the teachers agree on *some* things to avoid confusion among learners? Why do three different GI attendings have three different opinions on how to approach a patient with an upper GI bleed? Should we hang both IV drips of proton pump inhibitor and IV Sandostatin or not? Should we order an urgent endoscopic procedure to find the source of acute bleeding or not? Should we check hemoglobin every four hours, six hours, twelve hours, or once a day? Should we perform the endoscopy on an outpatient basis and send the patient home? And what if all three GI attendings agree on the same thing? Does that suggest that the decision was the correct one? If so, would such actions be based on experience or evidence?

As doctors, how many of us were practicing cost-effective medical care during our training? As patients or consumers, how many of us think health care is too expensive? Fortunately, today there are other square pegs like me who are asking similar questions. This has led to such campaigns as the American Board of Internal Medicine's Choosing Wisely. Unfortunately, back then, I didn't have much support for the questions I asked, especially from other academicians who were raised in ivory towers and still called these towers their home. I was still young and naïve. Intent was always the only thing that mattered to me, and I wore it as proudly as the ID badges of my children.

As I've grown older, though, I have learned—although I dislike it—that perception is the only thing that matters. As I continued to demand old school excellence and constant evidence to support decisions, I stuck out like my powder blue LaDainian Tomlinson jersey in the black hole section of an Oakland Raiders game (another story for another time.) As a result, I ticked off a lot of homer fans—I mean attendings. My goal was not to call anyone out, but to get "they" to understand that this was about "us." We were responsible for educating the doctors of tomorrow. We needed to allow independence so that the residents could grow. However, such freedom needed to be balanced by equal parts experience and evidence.

As you may imagine, this was not a conversation anyone wanted to have. To allow such talk would mean that we needed to improve the education of our teachers. Long before I learned to keep my mouth closed at departmental meetings, I suggested that all academic attendings on teaching services should have a mandatory in-service exam every year just like the residents-in-training. If we failed the exam, how exactly could we be considered qualified to teach residents? Would patients want a doctor to take care of them if they knew that the doctor had failed multiple attempts to pass the board certification exam? Although I still believe I was right, I wish I had kept these thoughts to myself. Why? Unfortunately, once perceptions become reality, no one—not even in academic medicine, where we were supposed to look for firsthand evidence and examine the data ourselves—would care about the intent.

Although my reputation with patients and learners was moving in a positive direction, my relationships with my colleagues, with few exceptions, were headed in the wrong direction. I was too naïve and too stubborn to realize that both sides needed to change. The failure of effective communication, like my famous drawing as a second-year resident, reflects crap falling downstream from high above. Sadly, I was focused on HOPESDREAMS when I should have known that the future would bring much more FEARSTEARS.

63

Reflective Notes

Attaining wisdom while creating confusion

I had been at LBJ for so long that I could actually go back and look at notes I had written as a medical student. Reflecting on my notes, I realized that I had changed, perhaps best illustrated by T.S. Eliot: "Where is the life we have lost in living, where is the wisdom we have lost in knowledge, where is the knowledge we have lost in information?"

As a medical student, everything around me represented information in the form of disjointed facts. One patient to the next, one exam to the next, one disease to the next. If a patient informed me that his teeth hurt when he urinated, I would've actually presented the information on rounds, and sadly, the attending may have "agreed with above." During residency, the information was slowly getting compartmentalized into knowledge that was guided more by experience than evidence. I could now ask the question "do your teeth sometimes hurt when you urinate?" If the answer was "yes," I could reasonably assume that the value of the history would be limited because the answer to multiple questions, regardless of the questions' ridiculousness, would certainly be "yes."

Ah, knowledge is better than information. Something was still missing, though, and that came with the transition to being an attending. (You can call me a pretending if you like, but I prefer wise pretending.) Now I could actually use the aforementioned ridiculous question as a problem related to a positive review of system (when the patient answers yes to all questions and everything is wrong and everything hurts). The wisdom allowed me to think about why the answer was "yes" to such a ridiculous question. Was there a language barrier? Was there an educational barrier? Was there an understanding barrier? Was there an underlying psychiatric disorder or a primary or secondary involvement of the central nervous system that may be infectious, metabolic, vascular, or perhaps related to nutrition or polysubstance abuse? How about Wilson's or Whipple's? Porphyria? Vasculitis? Chronic lead poisoning?

For years, I was proud of myself. I had finally attained wisdom and my notes reflected a broad differential diagnosis. Unlike others, I was able to clinically narrow such a differential based on pretest probability. This allowed me to provide cost-effective care to all my patients. In time, LBJ reminded me that this was not enough. I actually wanted to know the whys beyond the academic answers. The results were reflected in my notes that still summarized the evidence-based differential diagnosis and cost-effective analysis leading to effective treatment. However, the notes were now speaking to those who were reading, hoping someone was listening, just like my patients hoped that their doctor was listening. I must admit that I too was guilty of not listening for years. Here are some of my notes:

"Do we really understand why she is noncompliant with her medications?"

"Perhaps the history of present illness began in her childhood. Were there circumstances that led to the choices that she made, including substance abuse?"

"His eyes tell the rest of the story. I wish I could give him a hug and never let go."

"It has been close to two weeks in the hospital and there has not been a single visitor for this patient."

I often wonder how my thought process would have been different if I hadn't spent over a third of my life to date at a county hospital. What one knows, one sees. I have seen, over the years, the lives of my patients as if they were my own family members. And in doing so, in spite of our cultural differences and economic backgrounds, I have seen the common thread of HOPESFEARSDREAMSTEARS.

64

Laughter

An overlooked teaching tool

Not all notes were philosophical, and although I was changing, rounds were still about tough love. Spontaneous bouts of unexpected consequences were always welcomed and necessary for my survival at LBJ. One particular occurrence remains firmly entrenched in my mind as if it took place yesterday. We had started post-call rounds at 6:00 a.m. and had admitted sixteen new patients overnight. As a result, we did not physically see the sixteenth patient until around 11:30 a.m. This patient reflected all of the Mehta-isms that I could think of (see next page).

The patient, who was the last admission on that particular call day, presented with nausea, vomiting, and diarrhea. He also reported some nonspecific weight loss. The residents had diagnosed him with gastroenteritis. They were confident of their diagnosis because the CT scan of the abdomen was negative (I call the CT scan the fifth vital sign in the emergency room and the reason all our patients will be glowing in the dark several decades from now). The labs were "nonspecific" and "unremarkable," according to the residents. The patient was treated with IV fluids and medications to control his nausea and vomiting while his stool was sent for

MEHTA-ISMS

1) The last admission will always be the sickest.

2) The residents are tired by the last admission and, unless the labs or imaging studies from the emergency room were abnormal, will likely and erroneously think that the patient is "stable."

3) When stable patients become unstable, the residents likely missed something on the physical exam.

4) When the shit hits the fan, I will be looking for "they," since according to the residents, "they didn't tell me this" and "they missed it at the other hospital."

5) William Shakespeare asserted "Let every eye negotiate itself and trust no agent." When the residents are tired, even the most obvious findings will be overlooked. NNN was once presented a patient that was a white man but when he went to examine the patient, he turned out to be a black man.

6) The sickest patient never speaks English, a common issue at LBJ.

7) Residents will probably tell me about rule number six as an excuse and follow-up with "we tried but couldn't find a translator."

8) Fever is a reflection of inflammation, not infection, and the same rule applied to an elevated white blood cell count.

9) Look at the patient first and labs second.

10) The only time the last admission is stable is when I try to round on them first, assuming the worst.

cultures. When I walked into the room, the patient was obviously short of breath.

"He has diarrhea, Dr. Mehta, and secondary metabolic acidosis. He is just trying to blow off the excess acid."

"What else could it be?" I asked.

Silence.

"Did you get a chest x-ray or think about cardiopulmonary pathology?"

Silence.

The diagnosis was becoming more obvious as I approached the patient. He had a visibly enlarged thyroid gland, known as goiter. I placed my stethoscope over the thyroid gland and heard a bruit. His eyeballs looked as if they would pop out of their sockets. As such, he had exophthalmos. Examination of his legs revealed the presence of pretibial myxedema.

"Yes, we saw that, Dr. Mehta, but he had diarrhea and you told us before that African American patients may have exophthalmos-like features that don't necessarily reflect thyroid disease. Besides, he has gastroenteritis."

I had already asked the team if they had found anything abnormal on the physical exam and the answer was a collective "no." What one knows, one sees, and sadly since most pretendings are blind to the physical exam, by extension so are the residents.

The nurse walked in and told us that she placed the patient on oxygen because "his oxygen saturations have been dropping." The patient had a tremor when his arms were extended, and his reflexes were exaggerated and symmetric. As the events unfolded, I was turning from my light shade of brown to dark brown.

"You found nothing on his exam, and yet he has Graves' disease!" I started to examine the heart, and grew increasingly concerned about congestive heart failure. "How much fluid are you giving this man?"

"They gave him two liters of fluids in the emergency room and we gave him another two liters because his heart rate was not coming down and he has gastroenteritis so he is volume depleted."

"This man is in thyroid storm! Did you not calculate his Burch-Wartofsky score? Of course not, because you didn't even think he had thyrotoxicosis! Storm is acute but most thyrotoxicosis is chronic. Why is that important?"

Silence.

"Because the heart has been remodeling for years due to excessive metabolic demand and the patient may have congestive heart failure." We calculated his score and the patient was in storm. "Stop the fluids, start a beta blocker, call endocrinology now, get an echo, and begin PTU or Methimazole!"

I couldn't think of anything else to say and by now was pissed off. "God damn it, this patient is crapping out, transfer him to the MICU now!"

The patient was found to be in thyroid storm with severe congestive heart failure and an ejection fraction of less than 10% with four-chamber dilation on the echocardiogram. He survived in spite of us not because of us. Thanks to the combined efforts of the endocrinology, cardiology, and MICU teams, the patient was discharged home in stable condition.

How could such a stressful situation have been humorous? I failed to mention that the intern on my team had been in a research lab for over five years. During this time, he had no direct patient contact and spoke very little English. Therefore, his clinical experience was clearly lacking, and yet he was responsible for writing the transfer note to the MICU. I received a phone call from the MICU attending about thirty minutes after the patient was transferred. I was assuming that the patient was not doing well, but the MICU attending's laughter reassured me. "So why are you calling me?" I asked, dumbfounded.

"Let's just say that you need to be careful with the literal, I mean literal interpretation of what you say on rounds," he said, stopping often between his words to control his laughter.

"Huh?" I was confused.

"Just read the brief, and I mean brief transfer note."

"I don't understand. My intern has already finished the transfer note? It's been less than thirty minutes. I think that has to be a new record."

"Just read the transfer note and you'll understand." He was still laughing as he hung up the phone.

We were still in the era of paper trails, so I went to the MICU to look at the chart. This was the transfer note from my intern: "Dr. Mehta says the patient is crapping out, will transfer to MICU!!!!" I had to read it several times to make sure that my eyes were not deceiving me. I kept flipping back and forth for the rest of note, but that was it. That was the complete transfer note! I heard laughter behind me and saw the MICU team, including the attending. I started to laugh myself, and a moment of tension was gone in a second.

I later discussed the note with the intern and helped him to understand the error of his ways. I even shared a personal example of how I'd been told in the past that the medical record was not a Danielle Steel novel and that exclamation points should be avoided. He started laughing. When I asked him why, he told me he had friends in China who read Danielle Steel. By now, I had joined in the laughter. I told him about how I'd once forgotten to tell an attending during medical school that the patient had a pulmonary embolus overnight during my presentation. I told him about my tilt story from medical school and he couldn't stop laughing. I still may change the tone of my voice during rounds, although knowing the unintended consequences of my words, I'm extremely careful in choosing my words now. Perhaps Patch Adams was right: Laughter is the best medicine. If patients can have dental pain due to micturition, than why can't doctors HOPE to "crap out" from laughter that leads to uncontrollable TEARS.

Every destination has a journey, and every journey has a story. By now I had probably seen over 25,000 patients and trained over 1,000 students and residents. Over the years, patients would present with similar diseases with some subtleties, like questions on a board exam. After having spent a decade in academia, on the surface, all patients and diseases were starting to look the same. Our mind seemed to be repeating the same story. "Here is yet another admission for recurrent uncontrolled blood pressure and diabetes mellitus. Let's artificially and transiently fix the numbers, and send the patient home before the next one shows up."

However, what made each patient encounter memorable, especially when surrounded by learners, was "the rest of the story" that even Paul Harvey would have been proud of. I always looked for laughter, since if I couldn't heal patient suffering—or stop the students and residents from suffering on my rotation—at least somehow we could share a moment "crapping out" together.

Another similar incident involved a patient who reportedly had altered mental status in the emergency room. We had all been taught to perform the mini-mental status exam on such patients to determine the level of cognition. As an educator, I would attempt to demonstrate different portions of the exam at the bedside while talking to and examining the patient. I had already asked questions related to orientation and registration, and no issues were present. Next came questions to gauge attention and calculation. I asked the patient to spell *world*. He responded, "W-O-R-L-D."

"Very good," I said. "Now spell it backwards."

He paused for a moment and started, "T-I . . . ."

There was a smile on his face. I thought he misunderstood my question, so I asked him again. "My apologies sir, but perhaps you misunderstood my question. I would like for you to spell *world*."

He did so, so I asked him again to spell it backwards. With a deadpan expression he started again, "T-I . . . ."

By now the residents were laughing. Suddenly IT hit me! I had asked him to spell IT backwards. The joke was on me.

"I got you, Doc, didn't I!" said Mr. World. That was the end of my mini-mental status exam on that patient, but I learned a valuable lesson that I shared with my learners moving forward: laugh at yourself, and others will always join in.

Now I understood why NNN told us so many stories. His intent was to make us better, but in our younger days, we saw him as Walter Matthau in *Grumpy Old Men*. Over the years, I had turned into Grumpy Young Man. Maybe that's why they called me NNN, Jr. So I changed the theme of my stories. To remind learners that doctors are humans, I talked about how I missed something as a student or resident. More importantly, my stories kept them well-rounded by involving humor. In doing so, we would share a new bond, and their preconceived notions of me would change.

The new conversations were always unrehearsed and unintentional. The team had once admitted a patient with a lower GI bleed who needed an inpatient colonoscopy to determine the cause and appropriate interventions. I reminded the team that when I was a resident at LBJ, there was a GI Fellow named Dr. Colon. Everyone started chuckling. I told them about a neurosurgeon named Dr. Megahead. By now, other doctors and patients in the emergency room were looking at our group, because the laughter had turned into an uproar.

The student, who seldom spoke a word, chimed in, "There was a doctor in my hometown who was an OB/GYN by the name of Dr. Beaver."

Tears were forming in our eyes and I thought we were all headed for *globus hystericus* when the lead resident continued, "I would say you're making that up but there was a urologist—and I confirmed it through the Yellow Pages—his name was Dr. Richard Chop."

By now we must have sounded like a group of hyenas because the ER attending came over to ask us what was so funny and if everything was ok. Before I could answer, the resident continued, "Dr. Chop, however, went by another preferred first name."

To prevent myself from collapsing on the floor, I actually had to brace myself on the intern's shoulder for support. We repeated the story to the ER attending, who had turned completely red and had tears in his eyes from the laughter. He called his team over and shared the story with his group. Lost in all the commotion were the patients around us, all of whom were laughing, including the patient who had presented with the lower GI bleed.

I knew that I had succeeded at multiple levels when I pulled the curtain to talk to the patient. "Doc, I gotta tell you. I was nervous about the procedure y'all are planning this morning to help me, but after listening to you guys, I feel better already. Shoot, I thought I was gonna bust a gut hearing you guys with all those funny names." He realized what he said, and the hysterical laughter started all over again. HOPESFEARSDREAMSTEARS may come and go, but laughter shared with others is a moment that lasts forever.

65

Beginning of End

Broken heart and soul

Although I was a big fan of Pink Floyd, I refused to get comfortably numb. It was very difficult to maintain high educational standards, and as such I stuck out like a sore thumb. The frontline troops with whom I had built relationships over the years, including students who were now junior faculty members, nurses, patients, ancillary staff, and anyone who felt as if they belonged somehow at The County, understood my intentions.

Unfortunately, I could not undo the perceptions that had been created in the minds of my bosses. The pillar of all human relationships is effective, open-ended communication, be it doctor-patient, husband-wife, father-daughter, teacher-student, or boss-employee. I had slowly and effectively succeeded at every type of relationship, except for the latter. I was focused on intention but my boss only cared about perception. (Ah, the wisdom of age. If it could only come in a gift-wrapped box at an earlier time in life to accompany the energy of youth). Band-Aid diplomacy, especially when it's not mutual, always fails, and the writing on the wall was visible enough for a blind man to see. I would be leaving LBJ, a place that meant everything to me.

HOPESFEARSDREAMSTEARS would be left unfinished. A poem that I had written, titled LBJ, was suddenly playing in a continuous loop in my head (see box on next page).

I was a flood of emotions and questions, both rational and irrational. How could this happen? Why did this happen? This isn't happening! Should I just go back and teach high school English? Will I find another job? What will my kids and wife think of me? I was completely broken and it was still three months before I would leave. I could not eat, sleep, or think straight. My sugars were out of control (yes, I'm a diabetic) and suddenly I was popping the purple pill known as Nexium twice a day. I literally felt as if I was dying, and the pain in my heart was there twenty-four hours a day.

I had always said tongue-in-cheek to the residents that "the eyes are windows to the soul if you are religious, but if you're Dr. Mehta, the eyes are the windows to systemic diseases including diabetes, hypertension, infections, vasculitis, cholesterol emboli, and even cancer." I had always hoped they would remember the latter, but when they looked into my eyes all they could see was a soul that was hurting. I had not told anyone of the eminent divorce except my family. Perhaps I was hoping against hope that it wouldn't happen. Perhaps I was just going through Kübler-Ross stages on my own. Hell, I didn't know what I was thinking—I was sleeping only two hours a day.

I still went to work every day, and the residents were quick to pick up on my nonverbal clues, including the Samsonite luggage that I carried under my eyelids. I had never been a good poker player and it showed. A group of them stopped by my office before clinic. I shut the door and started the conversation.

LBJ

You are my heart;
You are my soul;
You are my LBJ.

Full of passion;
Full of care;
Never complaining;
Life's not fair.

What makes her special?
You say
It's the people who do
As they say.

The motley crowd is full
Of different colors and creeds;
Somehow not having forgotten
The joy of sewing your own seeds.

I feel you as I drive up;
To start the day at 6:00 a.m.;
Smiling, a gentle tear forming
Why can't healthcare for all be the same?

You and I
Share a special bond;
For we cure with a hug, a handshake,
Our magic wand.

Donna, Bertha, Sandra, Kim;
My role models of "Service to humanity is service to Him."

Ironic in that doctors see you
As a means not an end;
Forgetting your role in the slippery ladder they ascend.

So another 40 years here
And with you I will die;
Having lived a fulfilled life
Never questioning my worthy or why.

Thank you LBJ
For all that you do
In your heartbeat
I feel all that is true.

"I think I know what this may be about, but you go first. I'm listening."

"Dr. Mehta, remember the quote you taught us about how the eyes are windows to the soul and by extension systemic diseases?"

I was already tearing up because residents had given me a handmade picture of the retina three years earlier. The quote accompanying the masterpiece was screaming back at me in silence.

"Yes. Go on." I tried to create some spit in my mouth so that I could swallow the lump in my throat.

"Well, we're hearing all kinds of rumors, but forget all the rumors because what we see is that your soul is hurting when we look into your eyes. Please tell us what is wrong and we're not leaving until you do."

There was so much that I wanted to say and so many fingers that I wanted to point, especially at "they." I could not get the words out of my mouth, but instead they came floating like pearls out of my eyes. I apologized for my awkwardness and told them that it was time for me to move on. I must have taught them well because they were taking turns firing back my own quotes between the sobs and twin lakes that were flooding their faces.

"You taught us that the wealth of a soul is measured by what it feels and its poverty is judged by what it doesn't. This is bullshit. We feel that we need to make this right. You're not going to leave us. Tell us details. Tell us who we can go talk to. We're going to start a petition. This is bullshit. Pardon my language but there's no other way for us to voice this. We'll do whatever it takes. We don't care. We've talked to lots of other people. We're all on the same page. We're not going to let this happen."

Ah, the energy of youth, I was thinking to myself. It was as if there was a mirror in front of me and I was looking at myself fifteen years earlier. Unfortunately, I had learned the consequences of perceptions becoming reality for the wrong reasons, and how no one cared about my intentions. I gathered my composure. I told them that if they cared for me that they would take no such actions. I didn't want them to make the same mistakes that I had made in burning invisible bridges, even with good intentions. I was concerned since many in the room were headed towards fellowship or still had years left in their residency training.

I explained to them about how I'd been wrong over the years and that they must balance intention with perception, and energy with wisdom. I reminded them not to compromise their value system. In the end all that mattered was their ability to heal with equal parts heart and mind, not only when it came to patients, but more importantly with all relationships in life. I told them that I was starting to preach again and as such felt old. Maybe they were correct, and I'd finally become their surrogate dad. I forced a smile and they did the same.

"But there's something you could do to help me," I said suddenly. Their eyes lit up. "I need you to give me a hug before you leave this room, and keep on smiling, for laughter really is the best medicine."

Like wet sponges squeezing each other, we melted for a moment in each other's embrace and our clothes became our Kleenex. They exited one by one, and I gently shut the door behind me, putting my head down on the pillow on my desk as it absorbed all my HOPESFEARSDREAMSTEARS.

66

Last Three Months

I am the patient and you are my doctor.

The last three months of life at LBJ were the most difficult months of my professional and private life. I would be leaving a place that had become my home, and more importantly, leaving behind family members that had become my heartbeat. There was so much more that I had hoped to accomplish. As I told NNN, I felt as if I was leaving a house I had been building, one brick at a time for twenty years, still unfinished.

I wanted to say so much, but words failed me. I hoped to convey my message with my eyes but alas was not able to complete a single exchange without tears forming. I had become an endless source of saltwater. To avoid sharing my hurt with others, over time, I subconsciously started to look a bit to the side and over the shoulder of those that I would be talking to. I still struggle to overcome that handicap even today. For some strange reason, Sting's words kept ringing in my ears except the lyrics were a bit off. I wasn't happy, so why was "I'm so happy that I can't stop crying, I'm drowning in my tears" blaring in my head?

I tried to maintain Osler's *aequanimitas*, but felt

defeated. The hardest part was unlocking the door to my office every day. I was overwhelmed by the memories that surrounded the walls and ceilings in my little 8 by 12 foot room. Over the years, it had become the shape of my heart. I felt as if I was in *Groundhog Day*, going to my own funeral every day for three months. *Nice to know you haven't lost your sick sense of humor, Niraj.*

A nervous smile would cross my face as I thought of a quote on my desk from one of my psych patients, who had become my friend: "You're just jealous because the voices talk only to me!" *Well, guess what my friend, now they were talking to me, too. I wonder what my serotonin levels are.* Let's see, that must be the academician voice. *See, I told you fibromyalgia, chronic fatigue syndrome, and irritable bowel syndromes were real!* Those must be the voices of my unhappy patients seeking revenge. I felt as if I needed an emergency voice to control all the other voices in my head. That voice was actually external, and it came by many different names over the next three months. Slowly Sting faded away, and was replaced by Gloria Gaynor's "I Will Survive."

I don't know exactly how I survived, but I did, thanks to what suddenly turned into a parade of psychiatrists knocking on my office door. The unending supply of the world's biggest SSRI pill of encouragement and love came from both likely and unlikely sources. It included medical students, interns, residents, patients, and colleagues as expected. However, I was surprised to see social workers, janitors, cafeteria workers, security personal, and radiology and EKG technicians. We would sit and talk about times gone by and laugh till we cried, sharing stories of triumph and heartbreak. We would talk about Mehta-isms, cheat sheets for my rounds that I didn't know existed, and how my accent seemed to become more "country-like Texan" the longer I talked to patients—which always amused them since I was born in India. Some conversations involved physical exam findings, blood smears, spun urine samples looking for red blood cell casts, and amazing cases such as leprosy and Kikuchi-Fujimoto syndrome. Others involved how "they" didn't think much of me until "they" saw my office, my ID badges displaying my kids' pictures, or my broken spirit at the end of family conferences which delivered the news of terminal diseases with poor prognoses.

There were so many stories that I'd forgotten and some that I'd never ever heard before. In those three months, I was reminded over and over again that somehow I mattered and that I wouldn't be forgotten. It was as if over the years at LBJ, the lives of others had somehow become my own. To be loved by those around you had always been my HOPE, and in those final three months of what seemed like never-ending heartbreak, I realized that my DREAM had come true. That dream would not die on my departure from LBJ.

67

My Last Day at LBJ

Memory burn of forever relationships

The day I had thought would never come had arrived. It was August 31, 2010, my official last day at LBJ. Ironically, my team was post-call that day, and I was scheduled to start post-call rounds at 6:00 a.m. as had been the routine for the last fourteen years. My resident asked if we could start rounds later that morning. When I'd responded "no" without understanding their reasons, I received a phone call from the chief medical resident. "Dr. Mehta, we have something small planned for you tomorrow morning, so please start rounds later." I agreed, thinking a small goodbye was perhaps the plan since it was my last day. I was wrong once again.

Nothing could have prepared me for my last day of celebration at LBJ. I walked into 3C to see a parade of residents and nursing staff standing next to a giant "Thank You" banner with my name on it.

"Don't you people understand how unstable plaques suddenly rupture in times of extreme emotional disturbance? How many times have I drawn that diagram for you on rounds? You're going to kill me!" I said, smiling.

"You've drawn it plenty of times, and don't worry, we have sublingual nitroglycerin ready just in case," quipped one of the residents as the rest laughed.

So began my journey of unstable angina on my last day at LBJ. We walked towards 3B, where more residents and nurses were waiting inside the conference room. A breakfast was waiting as I silently chuckled about the memory of egg drop soup from my days as a resident. I was suddenly suffering from Sjogren's. My mouth went dry. *Was there an association between Sjogren's and unstable plaques? Not now, voice, shut up!*

I was given two albums on my last day. The first contained pictures of my time at LBJ for the past twenty years. The second album was much smaller, approximately the size of a 5-by-7 index card. On the front cover was a quote that I had used over and over in training doctors:

"Heal the sick, comfort the dying, and never confuse one for the other."

Was there such a thing as pseudo-Sjogren's? Because my mouth was dry, but my eyes were clearly going to fail the test for wetness. Not now, voice! I opened the cover and inside the album flaps were individual index cards from everyone using the problem/diagnosis approach that I'd used to teach, having first been introduced to it by NNN over fifteen years ago. Each card was signed and one of the residents chimed in: "And, Dr. Mehta notice that it is legible, each line has less than five words, and there are no abbreviations." Everyone joined in the laughter.

We continued the walk to the fourth-floor playground, now joined by fellows from different subspecialties, some of whom had been my students at one time. I told one of them to get the TPA (tissue plasminogen activator—a clot buster used to treat heart attacks) ready since I was about to have a heart attack and we still didn't have a cardiac catheterization lab at LBJ. More laughter.

The sun was already out and we took more pictures. Heaven was really a place called LBJ. It was my turn to speak, and as someone who was never at a loss for words, I was completely mute. How could words ever express at that moment in time what I felt? After a silence of what seemed forever, I was able to muster the strength to convey my final thoughts.

"I think I was wrong when I told you over the years that the eyes are the windows to the kidneys and systemic diseases, because when I look at all of you today, I realize that the eyes are windows to your soul. And each and every one of you has a beautiful soul that I feel lucky to have known over the years. I'll never forget you and before I start crying once again, give me a hug on the way out and always remember to see the sunrise at least once a year with someone you love before the sunset years of your life."

One by one, I won the lottery ticket over and over for the next fifteen minutes, getting priceless hugs of a lifetime. HOPESFEARSDREAMSTEARS.

There was one more daunting task left for me to perform on August 31, 2010, one that I'd been dreading for the past three months. I knew I wouldn't be able to complete this on my own and had asked my dad to come help me. We started in the late afternoon one by one to remove HOPESFEARSDREAMSTEARS. We pulled out one painful thumbtack at a time, taking down all the pictures and drawings in my office that had become My Heart and My Soul Mehta.

My dad had always been my hero and role model, perhaps because I was an only child. We were very close, and this wasn't going to be easy for either one of us. He had been my biggest confidant, my greatest supporter, my most honest critic, and even my secretary, helping me scan by hand over five thousand articles that I had gathered in the file cabinets in my office. There was an inverse relationship between tears and words for the next two hours as we spoke not a single word and let the Niagara Falls on our faces do the talking. All the words of encouragement from students, interns, residents, fellows, nurses, and patients over the years all seemed to be screaming along with the artwork as we took each piece down. I reflected on the memories that I had stored away in a file folder in my brain over the last twenty years. Unlike the articles that I was constantly updating as medical research evolved, I would never be able to replace or update these memories. I had three months and perhaps a lifetime at a subconscious level to prepare for a moment like this, but then again, sometimes we're never ready to say goodbye.

I had written a poem called "Before and After," believing that there are perhaps ten events in our life in which we are one person before the event and a different person after the event. I had never imagined that this profoundly sad moment would be one of those events. Slowly and deliberately, my dad and I filled each cardboard box with the priceless treasures of my rectangular office that had become the shape of my heart. We loaded up the boxes in the trunk of his SUV and just like that, my twenty years at The County had come to an end. I told him that I needed just a few minutes, and even he looked dumbfounded at what he saw next.

I took one last unhurried serpentine walk through the LBJ parking lot, reflecting on my journey. When I was a third-year medical student, all I had wanted to be was a fourth-year medical student. After all, I didn't know anything as a third-year medical student. What was I good for? Patients liked me, but how was that going to help my evaluation from the attending? What about the board exams? Who cares if I watched TV with the patient or we shared jokes and food?

No, the fourth-year student was known as the "acting intern," and although they clearly seemed to be acting on certain days, at least the fourth-year students were better actors than I was. When I became an acting intern, I realized that I was still not good enough. I wanted to be the intern. After all, I was just "acting," but the intern seemed to have the part down, including all the buzz words and catch phrases that everyone admired.

As I continued down memory lane, taking gentle steps in my serpentine pathway at LBJ that one last time, the voice continued. When I'd become an intern, I wanted to be the resident. No more best supporting actor. I wanted to be the lead and was tired of crap rolling downhill and landing on me. Some wishes do come true, and as I became the lead resident, I wanted to be the attending. After all, even the word sounds cool. *Attending.* Yeah, yeah, I know all about "pretending," but that could apply to, hell, the entire human race, so let's stay focused here.

Yes, I was an attending. Respect, money, fame, and fortune all at once. The pinnacle of the journey. The final achievement. And here I was now in the present moment. I stopped and smiled as a tear of happiness rolled down my cheek. All I wished for in this moment was to be a third-year medical student all over again. I had come to The County over twenty years ago, wanting to change the world one life at a time. In trying to do so, The County changed the one person that was otherwise not capable of changing himself. I thought I was the teacher, but in time I became the student, and every single person I met at The County—patients, nurses, medical students, residents, janitors, cafeteria workers, EKG and radiology technicians, security personnel, and policemen—

became my lifelong teachers. More importantly, everyone at The County became my friend.

In that moment, I realized that my journey was not ending. It was just beginning. The road less traveled must be embarked upon more often. The temporary detour would continue elsewhere, perhaps down Highway 59 South to Highway 288 South Exit McGregor Drive, straight to the other county hospital known as Ben Taub. I had always taught students and residents that the heart pumps blood the same way no matter where you trained. I hope my heart would continue to pump the blood to my soul at Ben Taub. It had taken me nearly half of my life, but I had once again found my heartbeat. My journey was my destination. Mother Teresa was right when she stated, "In this life we cannot do great things. We can only do small things with great love."

I returned to the SUV and noticed the smile on my dad's face. Pseudo-Bell's palsy must be hereditary since I thought I was once again looking in the mirror. I flashed a nervous half-smile back. We exited the parking lot, listening to Hindi music, as was our ritual. He tended to queue up music based on the mood, and today was no exception. "Kal Ho Naa Ho" by Sonu Nigam was playing as we sang silently in our heads, watching the sunset settle over a place I had seen so many sunrises. HOPESFEARSDREAMSTEARS.

Acknowledgments

A very special thank you to Michelle Zhang for her artistic vision in helping guide and design the cover of the book.

Medical School Interview: Winning Strategies from Admissions Faculty

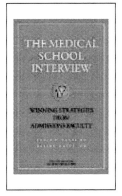

Samir Desai, MD and Rajani Katta, MD

ISBN # 9781937978013

The medical school interview is the most important factor in the admissions process. Our detailed advice, based on evidence from research in the field and the perspectives of admissions faculty, will provide you with the insiders' perspective.

How can you best prepare for the MMI, group interview, panel interview, and behavioral interview? What qualities would make applicants less likely to be admitted? What personal qualities are most valued by admissions faculty? What can students do to achieve maximum success during the interview?

This book shows medical school applicants how to develop the optimal strategy for interview success.

"…this is an extremely thorough handbook, covering the questions applicants are likely to be asked and the appropriate and inappropriate answers…likely to be found indispensable by readers embarking on the arduous process of applying to medical school."

- Kirkus Reviews

Medical School Scholarships, Grants & Awards: Insider Advice on How To Win Scholarships

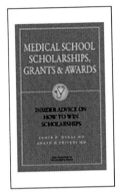

Samir Desai, MD and Anand Trivedi, MD

ISBN # 9781937978044

Residency match expert Dr. Samir Desai has helped students win medical school scholarships, grants, and awards, and now shares his perspectives in this new resource.

Over 500 awards are featured along with profiles of winners, proven strategies for success, and crucial tips. Learn how to craft a powerful scholarship application, write compelling essays, secure strong letters of recommendation, and stand out from the competition. Discover the best scholarships for you with awards for research, leadership, writing, global health, service, extracurricular activities, ethnicity, and gender.

Winners have reduced their medical school debt and strengthened their residency application, and see how you can too.

"The first 60 pages of this book are pure gold. It's filled with information about the application process, blunders to avoid, and nominating yourself to represent your school... The rest of the book, about 500 pages, consists of an excellent breakdown of scholarships with their descriptions...The book makes a complex process very simple."

- Helen (Amazon Review)

Success in Medical School: Insider Advice for the Preclinical Years

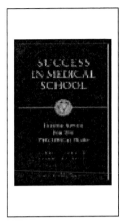

Samir P. Desai, MD and Rajani Katta, MD

ISBN # 9781937978006

According to the AAMC, the United States will have a shortage of 90,000 physicians by 2020. In the mid-1990s, the AAMC urged medical schools to expand enrollment. Class sizes have increased, and new schools have opened their doors. Unfortunately, rising enrollment in medical schools has not led to a corresponding increase in the number of residency positions.

As a result, medical students are finding it increasingly difficult to match with the specialty and program of their choice. "Competition is tightening," said Mona Signer, Executive Director of the National Resident Matching Program. "The growth in applicants is more than the increase in positions."

Now more than ever, preclinical students need to be well informed so that they can maximize their chances of success. The decisions you make early in medical school can have a significant impact on your future specialty options.

To build a strong foundation for your future physician career, and to match into your chosen field, you must maximize your preclinical education. In *Success in Medical School*, you'll learn specific strategies for success during these important years of medical school.

"Overall, I recommend this book...The book has so much information about everything that there has to be a part of the book that will satisfy your interests."

- Medical School Success website

Clinician's Guide to Laboratory Medicine: Pocket

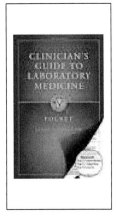

Samir P. Desai, MD

ISBN # 9780972556187

In this book, you will find practical approaches to lab test interpretation. It includes differential diagnoses, step-by-step approaches, and algorithms, all designed to answer your lab test questions in a flash. See why so many consider it a "must-have" book.

"In our Medicine Clerkship, the Clinician's Guide to Laboratory Medicine has quickly become one of the two most popular paperback books. Our students have praised the algorithms, tables, and ease of pursuit of clinical problems through better understanding of the utilization of tests appropriate to the problem at hand."

- Greg Magarian, MD, Director, 3rd Year Internal Medicine Clerkship, Oregon Health & Science University

"It provides an excellent practical approach to abnormal labs."

- Northwestern University Feinberg School of Medicine Internal Medicine Clerkship website.

"One of the best medical books of all time."

- The Medical Media Review

Success on the Wards: 250 Rules for Clerkship Success

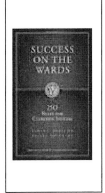

Samir P. Desai, MD and Rajani Katta, MD

ISBN # 9780972556194

This is an absolute must-read for students entering clinical rotations.

The authors of *The Successful Match: 200 Rules to Succeed in the Residency Match* bring their same combination of practical recommendations and evidence-based advice to clerkships.

The book begins as a how-to guide with clerkship-specific templates, along with sample notes and guides, for every aspect of clerkships. The book reviews proven strategies for success in patient care, write-ups, rounds, and other vital areas.

Grades in required rotations are one of the most important academic criteria used to select residents, and this critical year can determine career choices. This book shows students what they can do now to position themselves for match success. An invaluable resource for medical students - no student should be without it.

"*Success on the Wards* is an essential tool for the rising medical student...This book offers insider information on how a medical student can excel on the wards...I strongly recommend this book. It should be a must-read for any motivated student doctor."

- AMSA *The New Physician* (Review from September 2012)

"*Success on the Wards* is easily the best book I have read on how to succeed in clerkship. It is comprehensive, thorough and jam-packed with valuable information. Dr. Desai and Dr. Katta provide an all-encompassing look into what clerkship is really like."

- Review by Medaholic.com

The Successful Match: 200 Rules to Succeed in the Residency Match

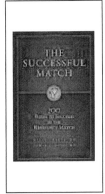

Rajani Katta, MD and Samir P. Desai, MD

ISBN # 9780972556170

What does it take to match into the specialty and program of your choice?

The key to a successful match hinges on the development of the right strategy. This book will show you how to develop the optimal strategy for success.

Who actually chooses the residents? We review the data on the decision-makers. What do these decision-makers care about? We review the data on the criteria that matter most to them. How can you convince them that you would be the right resident for their program? We provide concrete, practical recommendations based on their criteria.

At every step of the process, our recommendations are meant to maximize the impact of your application. This book is an invaluable resource to help you gain that extra edge.

"Drs. Rajani Katta and Samir P. Desai provide the medical student reader with detailed preparation for the matching process. The rules and accompanying tips make the book user-friendly. The format is especially appealing to those pressed for time or looking for a single key element for a particular process."

- Review in the American Medical Student Association journal, *The New Physician*

The Resident's Guide to the Fellowship Match

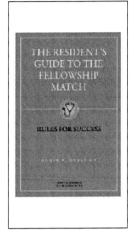

Samir P. Desai, MD

ISBN # 9781937978020

What does it take to match into the subspecialty and fellowship program of your choice?

Our detailed advice, based on evidence from research in the field and the perspectives of fellowship program directors, will provide you with the insiders' perspective.

What are criteria most important to decision-makers? What can you do to have the best possible letters of recommendation written on your behalf? How can you develop a powerful and compelling personal statement? How can you overcome the obstacles of residency to publish research? What can you do to achieve maximum success during the interview?

This book shows fellowship applicants how to develop the optimal strategy for success - an invaluable resource to help applicants gain that extra edge.

"Very detailed book to help you get fellowship position. The quotes from fellowship program directors are really helpful…it's like your own personal mentor full of great advice. Highly recommend this book."

- Ron (Amazon Review)

Connect with Niraj Mehta

► http://www.NirajMehtaMD.com/

► https://twitter.com/NirajMehtaMD

► https://www.facebook.com/pages/Niraj-Mehta-MD/297978113729349

MD2B Titles

The Medical School Interview: Winning Strategies from Admissions Faculty

Medical School Scholarships, Grants, & Awards: Insider Advice on How to Win Scholarships

Success in Medical School: Insider Advice for the Preclinical Years

Success on the Wards: 250 Rules for Clerkship Success

The Successful Match: 200 Rules to Succeed in the Residency Match

Resident's Guide to the Fellowship Match: Rules for Success

Clinician's Guide to Laboratory Medicine: Pocket

Available at www.MD2B.net

Bulk Sales

MD2B is able to provide discounts on any of our titles when purchased in bulk. For more information, please contact us at info@md2b.net or (713) 927-6830.